The Impact of Social Media on Public Health and Education

The Impact of Social Media on Public Health and Education

Guest Editor

Keren Dopelt

Basel • Beijing • Wuhan • Barcelona • Belgrade • Novi Sad • Cluj • Manchester

Guest Editor
Keren Dopelt
Public Health
Ashkelon Academic College
Ashkelon
Israel

Editorial Office
MDPI AG
Grosspeteranlage 5
4052 Basel, Switzerland

This is a reprint of the Special Issue, published open access by the journal *European Journal of Investigation in Health, Psychology and Education* (ISSN 2254-9625), freely accessible at: https://www.mdpi.com/journal/ejihpe/special_issues/V195I7K145.

For citation purposes, cite each article independently as indicated on the article page online and as indicated below:

Lastname, A.A.; Lastname, B.B. Article Title. *Journal Name* **Year**, *Volume Number*, Page Range.

ISBN 978-3-7258-7891-8 (Hbk)
ISBN 978-3-7258-7892-5 (PDF)
https://doi.org/10.3390/books978-3-7258-7892-5

Contents

About the Editor

Keren Dopelt

Keren Dopelt is an Associate Professor in the Department of Public Health at Ashkelon Academic College, Israel, where she holds tenure and serves in several academic leadership roles. Her research focuses on the sociology of health and illness, health promotion, and health inequalities, with a particular emphasis on the social and behavioral determinants of health. Her work addresses key contemporary challenges, including healthcare leadership, burnout among healthcare professionals, nutrition and mental health, and the impact of social media on public health. Prof. Dopelt is actively involved in international research collaborations and serves in global working groups in the fields of digital public health and health equity. She has received multiple awards for research excellence and was recognized with the Association of Schools of Public Health in the European Region (ASPHER) Early Career Excellence Award. In addition, she contributes extensively to the academic community as a reviewer, editorial board member, and Guest Editor of Special Issues in leading international journals.

Preface

The aim of this Reprint is to provide a comprehensive and interdisciplinary perspective on the complex relationships between social media, health, and education. The collected contributions examine key issues such as the dissemination of health information and misinformation, the influence of digital environments on mental health and well-being, and the role of social media in supporting or challenging learning processes. This Reprint is intended for researchers, practitioners, and policymakers working across the fields of public health, psychology, and education. By bringing together diverse approaches and empirical findings, it seeks to promote a deeper understanding of current challenges and to support the development of informed, evidence-based responses in an increasingly digital world.

Keren Dopelt
Guest Editor

European Journal of
Investigation in Health, Psychology and Education

MDPI

Editorial

The Impact of Social Media on Public Health and Education: Mechanisms, Vulnerabilities, and Policy Implications

Keren Dopelt

Department of Public Health, Ashkelon Academic College, Ashkelon 78211, Israel; dopelt@bgu.ac.il

1. Introduction

In the digital era, the line between evidence-based health information and viral misinformation has become increasingly blurred (Scheufele et al., 2021; Y. Wang et al., 2019). Health misinformation refers to false or misleading health-related claims shared without regard to scientific evidence, regardless of intent (Vraga & Bode, 2020). Social media platforms, while serving as an abundant source of information for billions worldwide, have simultaneously emerged as loci for the dissemination of misleading and inaccurate health content (Y. Wang et al., 2019; Tsao et al., 2021). Algorithm-driven content prioritization, centered on engagement rather than scientific validity, amplifies sensational narratives and facilitates the rapid spread of health misinformation (Feng et al., 2025). Empirical evidence suggests that false information diffuses significantly faster, deeper, and more broadly than truthful content on social networks, largely driven by novelty and emotional engagement (Vosoughi et al., 2018).

The widespread circulation of inaccurate health information across social media platforms constitutes a growing public health concern with tangible behavioral consequences. Exposure to misleading narratives has been associated with vaccination hesitancy, disordered eating patterns, body image dissatisfaction, excessive exercise behaviors, and the consumption of unregulated or potentially hazardous supplements (Pummerer et al., 2022). Beyond influencing individual choices, the high prevalence of health misinformation on social media may undermine evidence-based preventive behaviors and contribute to broader public health risks (Suarez-Lledo & Alvarez-Galvez, 2021).

In response to these challenges, the European Journal of Investigation in Health, Psychology and Education presents this Special Issue on "The Impact of Social Media on Public Health and Education." The contributions assembled herein not only examine the multifaceted relationship between social media and health behaviors but also critically explore the psychological, educational, and societal mechanisms underlying this phenomenon. By integrating interdisciplinary perspectives, this Special Issue seeks to advance scholarly dialogue and inform future research, policy, and practice. Understanding these dynamics requires examining the mechanisms through which social media actively shapes health behavior.

2. How Social Media Shapes Health Behavior

Social media platforms shape health behavior not only by increasing access to information, but by structuring how that information is encountered, interpreted, and trusted (Paul & Headley-Johnson, 2025). Platform personalization systems privilege visibility based on interaction metrics rather than epistemic quality, reinforcing certain narratives and fostering echo chambers in which repeated exposure enhances perceived credibility (Metzler &

Garcia, 2024). In such environments, emotionally charged, visually compelling, or sensational health messages are more likely to circulate widely than nuanced, evidence-based guidance (Carmona Pestaña et al., 2025).

Beyond platform-level amplification, the persuasive impact of health content is further shaped by how individuals cognitively process and evaluate information. Users frequently rely on heuristic cues, such as popularity metrics, perceived authenticity, and source attractiveness, when evaluating digital content, rather than systematically assessing scientific evidence (Metzger & Flanagin, 2013). Repeated exposure to similar claims may increase perceived accuracy through familiarity effects, strengthening belief even in the absence of empirical support (Pillai & Fazio, 2021).

In addition to cognitive heuristics, relational dynamics embedded in influencer culture further intensify persuasive effects. Influencers, often lacking formal healthcare training, frequently shape public perceptions of diet, exercise, vaccination, and medical treatments, sometimes more effectively than trained health professionals (Basch et al., 2025; L. Wang et al., 2024). Through parasocial relationships, audiences develop a sense of intimacy and trust, which enhances the persuasive impact. Health advice embedded within lifestyle content may therefore be adopted not because of demonstrated efficacy, but because it aligns with aspirational identities and perceived authenticity (Sokolova & Kefi, 2020).

Together, these structural, cognitive, and relational processes position social media not merely as a communication channel but as a commercialized behavioral health ecosystem (Tu & Li, 2024). Importantly, the same mechanisms that amplify misleading health narratives may also facilitate the dissemination of evidence-based guidance. Social media platforms have demonstrated potential to support health education, promote preventive behaviors, and enhance peer-to-peer support among individuals managing chronic conditions (Moorhead et al., 2013; Naslund et al., 2016). During public health emergencies, digital platforms have been used to rapidly communicate risk information and mobilize communities at scale (Paul & Headley-Johnson, 2025). Systematic reviews suggest that the impact of social media on health behaviors is neither uniformly harmful nor uniformly beneficial, but context-dependent and shaped by platform governance, content credibility, and user engagement patterns.

While social media platforms can disseminate evidence-based guidance, the structural logic governing visibility often prioritizes engagement over accuracy. Engagement-driven architectures are structurally misaligned with population health objectives, as they reward emotional intensity and novelty rather than epistemic reliability.

3. Vulnerable Populations and Amplified Risk

While social media influences health behavior across demographic groups, its effects are not distributed equally. Adolescents and young adults are particularly susceptible to the persuasive and normative power of digital health content. Developmental sensitivity to peer evaluation and identity formation increases vulnerability to social comparison processes, especially in visually driven platforms (Avci et al., 2025; Rounsefell et al., 2020). Exposure to curated body ideals, restrictive dietary trends, and extreme fitness regimens has been associated with body dissatisfaction and disordered eating patterns (Dopelt & Houminer-Klepar, 2025; Rounsefell et al., 2020).

Structural inequalities further shape digital vulnerability. Individuals with limited health literacy or reduced access to formal healthcare resources may also face elevated risk. Social media can become a primary source of health information, increasing exposure to misleading or oversimplified claims (Suarez-Lledo & Alvarez-Galvez, 2021). Research suggests that lower eHealth literacy is associated with greater difficulty distinguishing credibility from non-credible online health information (Milanti et al., 2025; Norman &

 https://doi.org/10.3390/ejihpe16030043

Skinner, 2006). In parallel, communities characterized by historical mistrust toward medical institutions may be more receptive to alternative health narratives circulating online, particularly when communicated through relatable influencers rather than institutional authorities (Dopelt et al., 2023; Jamison et al., 2020).

Individuals managing chronic conditions frequently turn to digital communities for support, experiential knowledge, and validation. While such engagement can enhance empowerment and coping (Naslund et al., 2016), it may also expose users to unverified treatments, anecdotal remedies, or anti-medical discourses. When personal vulnerability converges with algorithmic amplification and parasocial trust, misleading content may become especially compelling, particularly when it resonates with unmet needs or prior skepticism (Cinelli et al., 2021; Lewandowsky et al., 2017).

This commercialized behavioral ecosystem reflects broader commercial determinants of health operating within digital infrastructures. Beyond individual vulnerability, it is also necessary to consider the commercial determinants of health (CDoH) shaping digital environments. While social media is often discussed through the lens of individual choice, these platforms operate within business models that prioritize engagement as a primary commodity, frequently rendering health considerations secondary. In the digital economy, health-related content may function as a byproduct, whereas sustained user attention is the product. For industries promoting health-harming goods, such as ultra-processed foods, alcohol, or tobacco, social media provides highly targeted advertising infrastructures that can circumvent traditional regulatory safeguards. By leveraging detailed user data, commercial actors may identify and exploit psychological vulnerabilities, contributing to the normalization of behaviors detrimental to public health. In this sense, the "environment" in which health behaviors unfold is not only social or psychological but also commercial, structured by corporate incentives embedded within platform design (Gilmore et al., 2023). The attention economy itself increasingly functions as a determinant of health, shaping not only what information circulates, but which health norms become socially dominant. When engagement becomes the primary metric for value, visibility, and, by extension, perceived legitimacy, it may become decoupled from scientific credibility.

4. The Role of Health Professionals and Educators

As social media continues to shape how health information is interpreted and acted upon, the role of health professionals and educators within digital discourse has become increasingly consequential. Healthcare institutions and practitioners are already using social media for communication, education, and outreach (Moorhead et al., 2013). However, the accelerating circulation of health information, particularly misinformation, requires more deliberate and strategically designed engagement. In digital environments where visibility often influences perceived credibility, professional silence may allow misleading narratives to gain disproportionate influence (Chou et al., 2018). The transformation of health communication in the digital age has reached a point where disengagement carries tangible consequences.

Healthcare professionals possess the expertise necessary to contextualize risk, interpret scientific uncertainty, and translate complex findings into accessible guidance. Yet traditional communication models, grounded in institutional authority and formal dissemination channels, may be insufficient within fast-paced, algorithm-driven environments (Southwell et al., 2019). In environments structured to reward high-arousal emotional content, nuanced scientific communication struggles to compete with polarizing narratives (Cascini et al., 2022). Effective digital engagement requires not only accuracy but also clarity, relatability, and an understanding of platform dynamics. Bridging the gap between

https://doi.org/10.3390/ejihpe16030043

scientific rigor and digital communication norms is therefore essential for maintaining public trust (Larson, 2018).

Educational institutions also play a critical role. Integrating digital health literacy into curricula can equip individuals with the skills needed to evaluate online content, recognize persuasive techniques, and distinguish between evidence-based information and misleading claims (Dopelt et al., 2021; Milanti et al., 2025). Rather than framing social media solely as a risk environment, educational approaches can foster critical engagement and empower users to navigate digital health spaces responsibly.

At the policy level, coordinated strategies are required to address the structural drivers of misinformation. Recent regulatory initiatives, such as the European Union's Digital Services Act and the World Health Organization's infodemic management framework, reflect growing recognition of the need for greater transparency, platform accountability, and cross-sector collaboration in digital health governance. International public health bodies have emphasized the importance of infodemic management, transparency, and cross-sector collaboration in mitigating digital health risks (Briand et al., 2023; World Health Organization, 2020). Developing ethical guidelines for health-related content creation, promoting transparent disclosure practices among influencers, and strengthening accountability mechanisms for platform-driven amplification represent key workforce-level avenues for intervention (Bashkin et al., 2021). Such approaches may include graded content labeling for health claims and the downranking of demonstrably harmful misinformation within recommendation systems. They may also involve formalized collaborations with independent fact-checking initiatives, implemented with explicit safeguards for freedom of expression and due process. While regulation alone cannot eliminate misinformation, coordinated professional engagement and evidence-informed policy can mitigate its impact and reinforce public trust in health communication (Bashkin et al., 2022; Dopelt et al., 2023).

5. Implications for Research and Policy

Despite the expanding body of research, critical gaps remain in our understanding of how social media shapes sustained health behaviors and policy responses. While the prevalence of health misinformation and its behavioral correlates is well-documented, long-term causal pathways, cumulative exposure effects, and differential susceptibility across populations remain insufficiently understood. Longitudinal and experimental designs are needed to clarify how digitally mediated exposure interacts with psychological vulnerability to shape sustained health behaviors over time.

Research in this domain faces structural constraints. Rapid platform evolution, opaque recommendation systems, and limited data access restrict the ability to examine mechanisms of digital amplification. Without improved access to platform-level data and structured collaboration with technology companies, the development of targeted, evidence-based interventions will likely remain constrained.

Policy responses must therefore move beyond reactive regulation. Effective governance should promote transparency in sponsored health content, enforce clear disclosure standards for influencers, and address the amplification of demonstrably harmful misinformation, while safeguarding freedom of expression. Addressing these challenges requires coordinated engagement across public health authorities, policymakers, educators, researchers, and digital platform stakeholders.

These developments suggest that digital health communication stands at a regulatory and technological inflection point. The rapid integration of artificial intelligence (AI) into content production and recommendation systems introduces an additional layer of complexity. AI-generated health narratives, synthetic influencers, automated bot amplification, and increasingly personalized persuasive messaging may further blur the boundaries

 https://doi.org/10.3390/ejihpe16030043

between authentic expertise and algorithmically constructed authority. As generative technologies lower the barriers to producing credible-looking health content at scale, traditional markers of trustworthiness become more difficult to assess. This evolution intensifies the urgency of developing governance frameworks that address not only misinformation but the automation of persuasion itself.

6. The Role of This Special Issue—A Call to Action

This Special Issue of the European Journal of Investigation in Health, Psychology and Education serves as a platform for researchers, policymakers, educators, and healthcare professionals to critically examine the evolving relationship between social media and public health and education. As digital environments increasingly shape how health information is produced, disseminated, and consumed, coordinated scholarly engagement is essential.

By bringing together interdisciplinary perspectives, this Special Issue seeks to achieve the following:

1. Illuminate the mechanisms through which social media platforms influence health perceptions, norms, and behaviors.
2. Deepen the understanding of the psychological, social, and structural factors that contribute to the spread and persistence of health misinformation.
3. Examine the differential impact of digital health environments across populations, with particular attention to vulnerability and equity.
4. Inform the development of evidence-based communication strategies, educational frameworks, and policy responses.
5. Identify critical gaps in current knowledge and establish priorities for future research and cross-sector collaboration.

The articles included in this Special Issue reflect the multifaceted psychological and behavioral dimensions of social media engagement. Contributions examine how digital exposure shapes emotional processing, sleep patterns, depressive symptoms, body image, aggression, procrastination, loneliness, self-esteem, and vaccine uptake across diverse cultural contexts and age groups. Several studies explore mediating and moderating mechanisms, such as sleep disturbance, psychosocial vulnerability, and contextual influences, highlighting the complex pathways through which social media use translates into measurable health and educational outcomes. Together, these investigations underscore that social media is not merely a communication channel, but a psychologically active environment capable of influencing cognition, emotion, identity formation, and health-related behavior.

By fostering multidisciplinary dialogue, this Special Issue aims not only to analyze the challenges posed by social media but also to highlight its potential as a tool for responsible health promotion, for example, through digitally coordinated vaccination campaigns or online peer-support communities that demonstrably improve treatment adherence. Digital platforms are neither inherently detrimental nor inherently protective. Their public health impact ultimately reflects how they are governed, regulated, and engaged by institutions and users alike.

As algorithmic architectures increasingly shape access to health information, the responsibility to uphold evidence-based guidance extends beyond individual users to institutions, researchers, educators, and policymakers. Social media should no longer be conceptualized solely as a communication infrastructure, but as a powerful commercial determinant of health. The erosion of public trust may partly reflect structural features of digital business models that prioritize engagement-driven amplification over scientific nuance. Addressing the health consequences of digital environments, therefore, requires more than correcting isolated instances of misinformation; it requires sustained attention to

https://doi.org/10.3390/ejihpe16030043

platform governance, transparency, and accountability. As digital ecosystems continue to evolve through short-form formats, intensified personalization, and emerging AI-mediated content production, the governance of health information becomes increasingly complex. The future of public health will not be determined only in clinics and classrooms, but within algorithmic systems that govern attention, credibility, and collective perception. Failing to address this structural reality risks leaving population health subordinate to commercial logics of amplification.

Conflicts of Interest: The author declares no conflicts of interest.

References

Avci, H., Baams, L., & Kretschmer, T. (2025). A systematic review of social media use and adolescent identity development. *Adolescent Research Review, 10*(2), 219–236. [CrossRef]

Basch, C. H., Denholtz, C., Castillo, R. G., & Jaime, C. (2025). Public health in the age of TikTok: A content analysis of measles narratives. *International Journal of Infectious Diseases, 160*, 108055. [CrossRef]

Bashkin, O., Dopelt, K., Mor, Z., Leighton, L., Otok, R., Duplaga, M., MacLeod, F., De Nooijer, J., Neumark, Y., Paillard-Borg, S., Tulchinsky, T., Zelber-Sagi, S., & Davidovitch, N. (2021). The future public health workforce in a changing world: A conceptual framework for a European-Israeli knowledge transfer project. *International Journal of Environmental Research and Public Health, 18*(17), 9265. [CrossRef]

Bashkin, O., Otok, R., Leighton, L., Czabanowska, K., Barach, P., Davidovitch, N., Dopelt, K., Duplaga, M., Okenwa Emegwa, L., MacLeod, F., Neumark, Y., Raz, M. P., Tulchinsky, T., & Mor, Z. (2022). Emerging lessons from the COVID-19 pandemic about the decisive competencies needed for the public health workforce: A qualitative study. *Frontiers in Public Health, 10*, 990353. [CrossRef] [PubMed]

Briand, S., Hess, S., Nguyen, T., & Purnat, T. D. (2023). Infodemic management in the twenty-first century. In T. D. Purnat, T. Nguyen, & S. Briand (Eds.), *Managing infodemics in the 21st century: Addressing new public health challenges in the information ecosystem*. Springer. [CrossRef]

Carmona Pestaña, A., Herrera-Peco, I., Jiménez-Gómez, B., & Suárez-Llevat, C. (2025). Internet memes as drivers of health narratives and infodemics: Integrative review. *JMIR Infodemiology, 5*, e77029. [CrossRef]

Cascini, F., Pantovic, A., Al-Ajlouni, Y. A., Failla, G., Puleo, V., Melnyk, A., Lontano, A., & Ricciardi, W. (2022). Social media and attitudes towards a COVID-19 vaccination: A systematic review of the literature. *EClinicalMedicine, 48*, 101454. [CrossRef]

Chou, W. S., Oh, A., & Klein, W. M. P. (2018). Addressing health-related misinformation on social media. *JAMA, 320*(23), 2417–2418. [CrossRef]

Cinelli, M., De Francisci Morales, G., Galeazzi, A., Quattrociocchi, W., & Starnini, M. (2021). The echo chamber effect on social media. *Proceedings of the National Academy of Sciences of the United States of America, 118*(9), e2023301118. [CrossRef] [PubMed]

Dopelt, K., Abudin, A., Yukther, S., Shmukler, T., & Davidovitch, N. (2023). The association between levels of trust in the healthcare system and influenza vaccine hesitancy among college students in Israel. *Vaccines, 11*(11), 1728. [CrossRef]

Dopelt, K., Avni, N., Haimov-Sadikov, Y., Golan, I., & Davidovitch, N. (2021). Telemedicine and eHealth literacy in the era of COVID-19: A cross-sectional study in a peripheral clinic in Israel. *International Journal of Environmental Research and Public Health, 18*(18), 9556. [CrossRef]

Dopelt, K., & Houminer-Klepar, N. (2025). The impact of social media on disordered eating: Insights from Israel. *Nutrients, 17*(1), 180. [CrossRef] [PubMed]

Feng, X., Luo, J., Yang, Y., El Baz, D., & Shi, L. (2025). Health misinformation detection: Approaches, challenges and opportunities. *Inquiry: A Journal of Medical Care Organization, Provision and Financing, 62*, 469580251384784. [CrossRef]

Gilmore, A. B., Fabbri, A., Baum, F., Bertscher, A., Bondy, K., Chang, H. J., Demaio, S., Erzse, A., Freudenberg, N., Friel, S., Hofman, K. J., Johns, P., Abdool Karim, S., Lacy-Nichols, J., de Carvalho, C. M. P., Marten, R., McKee, M., Petticrew, M., Robertson, L., ... Thow, A. M. (2023). Defining and conceptualising the commercial determinants of health. *Lancet, 401*(10383), 1194–1213. [CrossRef]

Jamison, A. M., Broniatowski, D. A., Dredze, M., Wood-Doughty, Z., Khan, D., & Quinn, S. C. (2020). Vaccine-related advertising in the Facebook Ad Archive. *Vaccine, 38*(3), 512–520. [CrossRef] [PubMed]

Larson, H. J. (2018). The biggest pandemic risk? Viral misinformation. *Nature, 562*(7727), 309. [CrossRef] [PubMed]

Lewandowsky, S., Ecker, U. K. H., & Cook, J. (2017). Beyond misinformation: Understanding and coping with the "post-truth" era. *Journal of Applied Research in Memory and Cognition, 6*(4), 353–369. [CrossRef]

Metzger, M. J., & Flanagin, A. J. (2013). Credibility and trust of information in online environments: The use of cognitive heuristics. *Journal of Pragmatics, 59*(Pt B), 210–220. [CrossRef]

https://doi.org/10.3390/ejihpe16030043

Metzler, H., & Garcia, D. (2024). Social drivers and algorithmic mechanisms on digital media. *Perspectives on Psychological Science: A Journal of the Association for Psychological Science*, *19*(5), 735–748. [CrossRef]
Milanti, A., Norman, C., Chan, D. N. S., So, W. K. W., & Skinner, H. (2025). eHealth literacy 3.0: Updating the Norman and Skinner 2006 model. *Journal of Medical Internet Research*, *27*, e70112. [CrossRef]
Moorhead, S. A., Hazlett, D. E., Harrison, L., Carroll, J. K., Irwin, A., & Hoving, C. (2013). A new dimension of health care: Systematic review of the uses, benefits, and limitations of social media for health communication. *Journal of Medical Internet Research*, *15*(4), e85. [CrossRef]
Naslund, J. A., Aschbrenner, K. A., Marsch, L. A., & Bartels, S. J. (2016). The future of mental health care: Peer-to-peer support and social media. *Epidemiology and Psychiatric Sciences*, *25*(2), 113–122. [CrossRef] [PubMed]
Norman, C. D., & Skinner, H. A. (2006). eHealth literacy: Essential skills for consumer health in a networked world. *Journal of Medical Internet Research*, *8*(2), e9. [CrossRef]
Paul, B., & Headley-Johnson, S. A. (2025). The impact of social media on health behaviors, a systematic review. *Healthcare*, *13*(21), 2763. [CrossRef] [PubMed]
Pillai, R. M., & Fazio, L. K. (2021). The effects of repeating false and misleading information on belief. *Wiley Interdisciplinary Reviews: Cognitive Science*, *12*(6), e1573. [CrossRef]
Pummerer, L., Böhm, R., Lilleholt, L., Winter, K., Zettler, I., & Sassenberg, K. (2022). Conspiracy theories and their societal effects during the COVID-19 pandemic. *Social Psychological and Personality Science*, *13*(1), 49–59. [CrossRef]
Rounsefell, K., Gibson, S., McLean, S., Blair, M., Molenaar, A., Brennan, L., Truby, H., & McCaffrey, T. A. (2020). Social media, body image and food choices in healthy young adults: A mixed methods systematic review. *Nutrition & Dietetics: The Journal of the Dietitians Association of Australia*, *77*(1), 19–40. [CrossRef]
Scheufele, D. A., Hoffman, A. J., Neeley, L., & Reid, C. M. (2021). Misinformation about science in the public sphere. *Proceedings of the National Academy of Sciences of the United States of America*, *118*(15), e2104068118. [CrossRef]
Sokolova, K., & Kefi, H. (2020). Instagram and YouTube bloggers promote it, why should I buy? How credibility and parasocial interaction influence purchase intentions. *Journal of Retailing and Consumer Services*, *53*, 101742. [CrossRef]
Southwell, B. G., Niederdeppe, J., Cappella, J. N., Gaysynsky, A., Kelley, D. E., Oh, A., Peterson, E. B., & Chou, W. S. (2019). Misinformation as a misunderstood challenge to public health. *American Journal of Preventive Medicine*, *57*(2), 282–285. [CrossRef]
Suarez-Lledo, V., & Alvarez-Galvez, J. (2021). Prevalence of health misinformation on social media: Systematic review. *Journal of Medical Internet Research*, *23*(1), e17187. [CrossRef] [PubMed]
Tsao, S. F., Chen, H., Tisseverasinghe, T., Yang, Y., Li, L., & Butt, Z. A. (2021). What social media told us in the time of COVID-19: A scoping review. *The Lancet Digital Health*, *3*(3), e175–e194. [CrossRef] [PubMed]
Tu, C., & Li, X. (2024). Personal versus societal risk: Examining social media influence on individual and collective behaviors for COVID-19 containment. *Social Media + Society*, *10*(1), 1–14. [CrossRef]
Vosoughi, S., Roy, D., & Aral, S. (2018). The spread of true and false news online. *Science*, *359*(6380), 1146–1151. [CrossRef] [PubMed]
Vraga, E. K., & Bode, L. (2020). Defining misinformation and understanding its bounded nature: Using expertise and evidence for describing misinformation. *Political Communication*, *37*(1), 136–144. [CrossRef]
Wang, L., Li, X., Wang, D., & Zhu, J. (2024). Influence of social media fitness influencers' credibility on users' physical activity intentions. *Digital Health*, *10*, 20552076241302016. [CrossRef]
Wang, Y., McKee, M., Torbica, A., & Stuckler, D. (2019). Systematic literature review on the spread of health-related misinformation on social media. *Social Science & Medicine*, *240*, 112552. [CrossRef]
World Health Organization. (2020). *Managing the COVID-19 infodemic: Promoting healthy behaviours and mitigating the harm from misinformation and disinformation*. Available online: https://www.who.int/news/item/23-09-2020-managing-the-covid-19-infodemic-promoting-healthy-behaviours-and-mitigating-the-harm-from-misinformation-and-disinformation (accessed on 12 February 2026).

https://doi.org/10.3390/ejihpe16030043

European Journal of
Investigation in Health, Psychology and Education

MDPI

Article

Sleep Disturbance as a Mediator Between Problematic Social Media Use and Depressive Symptoms Among Mexican Undergraduate Nursing Students: A Multicenter Study

José Ángel Hernández-Mariano [1,†], Ana Cristina Castañeda-Márquez [2,†], Gledy Manuela Olmos-Rivera [3], Rocío Castillo-Díaz [4], Fani Villa-Rivas [4], Edith Araceli Cano-Estrada [5], Yaneth Citlalli Orbe-Orihuela [6], Miguel Trujillo-Martínez [7] and Monica Alethia Cureño-Díaz [8,*]

1 Department of Research, Hospital Juarez of Mexico, Mexico City 07760, Mexico
2 Scientific Research Institute, Juarez University of the State of Durango, Durango 34000, Mexico
3 Nursing School, Hospital Juárez de México, Mexico City 04510, Mexico
4 Faculty of Nursing and Midwifery, Juarez University of the State of Durango, Durango 34217, Mexico
5 Superior School of Tlahuelilpan, Autonomous University of the State of Hidalgo, Tlahuelilpan 42780, Mexico
6 Department of Chronic Infections and Cancer, Center for Research on Infectious Diseases, National Institute of Public Health, Cuernavaca 62100, Mexico
7 General Hospital with Family Medicine Unit Number 7, Mexican Social Security Institute, Cuautla 62740, Mexico
8 Department of Institutional Intelligence in Oncological Health, National Institute of Cancerology, Mexico City 14080, Mexico
* Correspondence: mcureno@facmed.unam.mx; Tel.: +52-5556280400 (ext. 71045)
† These authors contributed equally to this work.

Abstract: Background: Social media addiction is a growing concern among undergraduates, with nursing students particularly vulnerable as their stressful academic and clinical context may promote excessive use, impaired sleep, and higher depression risk. Therefore, we aimed to evaluate whether sleep disturbance mediates the association between problematic social media use and symptoms of depression among nursing students in Mexico. Methods: We conducted a multicenter, cross-sectional, analytical study using a random sample of 638 nursing students from three Mexican public universities. Between August and December 2024, participants completed validated scales for social media addiction, sleep quality, and depression. Counterfactual causal mediation analysis was performed using logistic regression with robust errors. Results: Sleep disturbance affected 51.7% of students, and 27.5% reported depression. Social media addiction showed a dose–response association with both outcomes. Mediation analysis revealed a total effect on depression (OR = 2.19; 95% CI = 1.45–3.30) and an indirect effect via sleep disturbance (OR = 1.22; 95% CI = 1.01–1.38), explaining 31.4% of the effect. Conclusions: Sleep disturbance partially mediates this association. Interventions addressing digital behavior and sleep hygiene may improve mental health in nursing students.

Keywords: social media addiction; depression; sleep disorders; nursing students

1. Introduction

Mental health disorders represent a significant challenge to global public health due to their high prevalence and profound impact. It is estimated that approximately one in eight individuals worldwide lives with a mental disorder (Fan et al., 2025), with depression being the most prevalent. Recent estimates suggest a global prevalence of depressive disorders of 3588.25 cases per 100,000 population (Zhang et al., 2024). In Mexico, it has been reported that 16% of young adults present with depressive symptoms, most of whom do not receive adequate care (Vázquez-Salas et al., 2023). This situation highlights the structural deficiencies of the mental health system, primarily due to the shortage of specialized services and the inequitable distribution of community and outpatient resources nationwide (Carmona-Huerta et al., 2021).

In this sense, undergraduate students are particularly vulnerable to developing mental disorders due to their constant exposure to academically and emotionally challenging environments. Factors such as academic overload, pressure to meet institutional expectations, peer competition, performance anxiety, and personal difficulties can act as chronic stressors that negatively affect their mental health (Liu et al., 2023; Mofatteh, 2020).

Among them, nursing students may be especially at risk of experiencing psychological distress due to the nature of their training. In addition to acquiring theoretical and technical knowledge, they are required to engage in clinical practice from the early stages of their education, often in emotionally intense and high-pressure environments. These include providing care for critically ill patients, witnessing human suffering, and facing death (Labrague et al., 2018; Silva et al., 2011). The emotional intensity of these experiences, which are uncommon in most other academic programs, may increase their susceptibility to anxiety, stress, burnout, and depressive symptoms (Consuelos-Sánchez et al., 2023; Hernández-Mariano et al., 2024; Sonmez et al., 2023; Vo et al., 2023). A recent meta-analysis estimated that, globally, approximately three in ten nursing students (29%) experience depression (Efstathiou et al., 2025).

Although depressive symptoms are also prevalent among students from other academic disciplines, nursing students face distinctive emotional and professional demands that differentiate them from the general college population (Akhtar et al., 2020). From the early stages of training, they are exposed to ethically challenging and emotionally charged situations linked to patient care—conditions rarely encountered in other academic programs. These experiences, combined with academic overload, irregular schedules, and clinical stress, may heighten their vulnerability to maladaptive coping behaviors, including excessive social media use and sleep disruption. Therefore, nursing students should not be regarded merely as representative of all university students but rather as a particularly sensitive subgroup within the health sciences, whose experiences may resemble those of other care-oriented disciplines such as medicine, psychology, or social work.

Currently, the study of emerging factors that could influence the mental health of undergraduate students has gained relevance, particularly the intensive use of social media (Salari et al., 2025). Social media addiction has been defined as a pattern of compulsive, uncontrolled, and persistent use of these platforms, which interferes with daily activities and generates significant distress when access is limited or interrupted (Amirthalingam & Khera, 2024). Although the evidence is still emerging, some studies suggest that this behavior could be related to sleep disorders (O. Ahmed et al., 2024).

Sleep disorders, defined as any alteration in the quantity, quality, or continuity of nighttime rest that compromises physical or psychological functioning during the day (Karna et al., 2025), have been associated with prolonged social media use; this association is particularly significant when social media use is concentrated at night (O. Ahmed et al., 2024; Alonzo et al., 2021). It has been suggested that factors such as screen time before bed, sustained emotional arousal, and difficulty mentally disconnecting from the digital environment may contribute to delayed sleep onset, frequent nighttime interruptions, or daytime sleepiness (Allen et al., 2018; Blume et al., 2019; Dresp-Langley & Hutt, 2022; Kinsella & Chin, 2024; Kumar et al., 2025). Nonetheless, the mechanisms underlying this possible relationship are not yet fully understood and may vary across individuals and contexts.

On the other hand, it has also been suggested that social media addiction could be associated with a higher likelihood of experiencing depressive symptoms. While several explanatory mechanisms have been proposed, such as negative social comparison, low self-esteem, or overexposure to emotionally intense content (M. Ahmed, 2023; Firth et al., 2024; Lițan, 2025; Samra et al., 2022), sleep impairment has been suggested as a possible mediator in this relationship. According to this hypothesis, problematic social media use may impair sleep quality, which in turn could disrupt neurotransmitter regulation and promote the secretion of proinflammatory cytokines, both mechanisms that have been implicated in the pathophysiology of depression (Dziurkowska & Wesolowski, 2021; Nicolaides et al., 2000; Nishuty et al., 2019). This interaction is especially relevant in university settings with high academic demands and unstable sleep routines.

Among nursing students, these conditions may be further exacerbated by the dual demands of theoretical instruction and practical clinical training, as well as by early exposure to emotionally taxing healthcare environments (Labrague et al., 2018; Silva et al., 2011). This issue becomes even more concerning given evidence suggesting that mental health problems that arise during undergraduate training often persist after students transition into the workforce (Rudman & Gustavsson, 2012). Nevertheless, few studies have simultaneously examined the relationship between social media addiction, sleep quality, and depressive symptoms in this specific population (AlAmer et al., 2020; Berdida, 2025). In the Mexican context, although these issues have been described individually (Bueno-Brito et al., 2024; Márquez-Ríos & Grimaldo-Zapata, 2024; Pérez et al., 2024; Vázquez et al., 2025), their interrelationships have been comparatively less explored. Investigating these associations may not only help to quantify the magnitude of the problem but also to identify potential targets for interventions aimed at promoting the well-being of future nursing professionals.

Recent global research has consistently demonstrated that excessive social media use is associated with sleep disturbances, depressive symptoms, and burnout among university students (Alimoradi et al., 2019; Corke et al., 2025; Osman, 2025; Yu et al., 2024). However, empirical studies examining these mechanisms in Latin American settings remain scarce, particularly among health sciences students. Although the biological and psychological mechanisms linking social media use, sleep disturbances, and depressive symptoms are considered universal, primarily involving circadian rhythm disruption, dopaminergic reward dysregulation, and the bidirectional relationship between sleep and mood (Levenson et al., 2017; Scott et al., 2021), their expression may vary across educational and social environments. In Mexico and other countries in the region, undergraduate students and clinical interns in health sciences represent an essential component of the healthcare workforce, often assuming patient care responsibilities during their training (Hernández-Mariano et al., 2024; Pan American Health Organization, 2025; World Health Organization, 2020).

This dual academic and clinical role exposes them to irregular schedules, emotional stress, and reduced sleep opportunities, conditions that may intensify the effects of problematic social media use on mental health. Expanding the evidence base in these populations is crucial to assess the external validity of current models and to design contextually relevant interventions that promote mental well-being among future healthcare professionals.

Therefore, we evaluated the association between problematic social media use, sleep disturbance, and depressive symptoms in undergraduate Mexican nursing students, testing a conceptual model in which sleep disturbance mediates the relationship between problematic social media use and depressive symptoms.

2. Materials and Methods

2.1. Design and Study Population

We conducted a multicenter, analytical, cross-sectional study among undergraduate nursing students in Mexico. The study population consisted of 1388 students enrolled in nursing training programs at three public universities located in Mexico City, Hidalgo, and Durango, between August and December 2024. The minimum sample size required for this study was calculated using the formula for relative measures of association (i.e., odds ratio) (Cvetković-Vega et al., 2021). We determined a sample size of 638 participants to estimate an odds ratio of at least 1.7, based on the following assumptions: a global prevalence of social media addiction among undergraduate students of 18.4% (Salari et al., 2025), a statistical power of 80%, and a 95% confidence level. Participants were selected using proportional stratified sampling by study site (Mexico City, Hidalgo, and Durango). Study participants were men and women aged 18 years or older. Pregnant women and students who were undergoing treatment with psychiatric medication at the time of the survey were excluded from the study.

2.2. Data Collection

General information was obtained through a structured questionnaire that included questions on the sociodemographic characteristics of the nursing students (i.e., sex, age, marital status, family monthly income, offspring, employment, and parental schooling); academic information (i.e., year in nursing program and scholarship); regular tobacco and alcohol consumption (i.e., current consumption greater than or equal to once per week); and we also obtained information on the frequency of social media utilization.

The problematic use of social media was assessed using the Social Media Addiction Scale-Student Form (SMAS-SF) (Sahin, 2018), which has been previously validated in the Mexican population (Valencia-Ortiz & Cabero-Almenara, 2019) and demonstrated acceptable internal consistency (Cronbach's alpha = 0.93). The SMAS-SF consists of 29 items organized into four dimensions and rated on a five-point Likert scale. (0, hardly ever; 1; 2, Sometimes; 3, Almost always). The SMAS-SF's scores range from a minimum of 29 to a maximum of 145. The ut-off points for classifying the level of problematic social media use are the following: 29–51, no addiction; 52–74, mild dependence; 75–97, moderate dependence; and >98, high dependency.

The Pittsburgh Sleep Quality Index (PSQI), which evaluates overall sleep quality over the past month, was used to assess sleep disturbance. The PSQI comprises 19 items grouped into seven subscales: self-reported sleep quality, sleep latency, sleep duration, habitual sleep efficiency, sleep disturbances, use of sleeping medication, and daytime dysfunction. Each of them is scored on a scale from 0 to 3, and the total global score is obtained by summing the component scores, yielding a range from 0 to 21. Higher scores indicate poorer sleep quality. A global PSQI score ≥ 5 indicates poor sleep. The PSQI has been previously validated in undergraduate students, demonstrating acceptable internal consistency (Cronbach's alpha = 0.78) (Ojeda-Paredes et al., 2019).

For depressive symptoms screening, we employed the straightforward seven-item shortened version of the Center for Epidemiologic Studies Depression Scale (CESD-7). This version, previously validated in the Mexican population, shows acceptable internal consistency (Cronbach's alpha > 0.83). The CESD-7 consists of 7 items and uses a 4-point Likert-type response scale. The total score, calculated by summing the item responses, ranges from 0 to 21. A score of 5 or higher indicates the presence of depression (Salinas-Rodríguez et al., 2014).

At each participating institution, students were invited through classroom announcements and institutional communication channels. Those who agreed to participate received detailed information about the study's objectives, voluntary nature, and confidentiality safeguards. After providing written informed consent, participants completed the self-administered questionnaire in supervised classroom sessions to ensure standardized conditions and to prevent discussion among participants. The average response time was approximately 20 min. All questionnaires were collected anonymously and coded to preserve participant confidentiality.

2.3. Statistical Analysis

The study variables were described using frequencies and percentages for categorical variables. We compared the general characteristics of the participants according to their sleep disturbance and depression status using the Pearson Chi-square test. The associations between social media addiction, sleep disturbance, and depression were evaluated using logistic regression models for each independent variable. The dose–response relationships between interest variables were also assessed in all models (a trend value of $p < 0.05$ was considered significant) (Patino & Ferreira, 2016).

Because sleep disturbance is a known risk factor for mood deterioration, we explored its mediating effect in the pathway connecting problematic social media use with depressive symptoms. To facilitate this analysis, we collapsed the last three categories of the "social media addiction" variable, thereby dichotomizing it into two strata: "no addiction" and "some degree of addiction." We then conducted a mediation analysis using binary exposure and mediator variables (Rijnhart et al., 2023). In our study, we utilized Stata's "mediate" command, a key tool in the counterfactual mediation model (Hicks & Tingley, 2011). This model, also known as the potential outcomes approach, is instrumental in decomposing the total effect of an exposure on an outcome into its direct and indirect components through a mediator (Byeon & Lee, 2023). We specified logistic models for the mediator (sleep disturbance) and the outcome (depression), both dichotomous. To ensure the robustness of our findings, we conducted a sensitivity analysis using the bootstrap method with 1000 replications (Jung, 2021). The consistency of the results with those of the original model validated our approach, leading us to report the effects estimated from the "mediate" command, expressed as odds ratios (OR) using the "stat or" command. Furthermore, we presented the percentage each effect (direct and indirect) represents relative to the total effect, aiding interpretation of the relative magnitude of each pathway.

To assess the robustness of the findings and verify whether the classification of social media addiction influenced the mediation results, we conducted a sensitivity analysis using an alternative grouping of the exposure variable. In this additional model, the categories no addiction and mild addiction were combined into a single reference group, while moderate and severe addiction were merged to represent problematic use. This reclassification aimed to explore whether the observed associations were consistent when using a broader definition of social media addiction. The mediation analysis was repeated using this dichotomized classification, with the same counterfactual framework, model specifications, and bootstrap procedure described above.

All models were adjusted for confounding factors. The selection of confounders for inclusion in the models was based on directed acyclic graphs (DAGs) (Cañón-Montañez & Rodríguez-Acelas, 2019; Digitale et al., 2022; Tennant et al., 2021). Age, sex, year of study in the nursing program, paid work, family monthly income, study site, family history of mental illness, and parental education were identified as the minimal sufficient adjustment set for the association between social media addiction and depression (Supplementary Figure S1). Variables not selected by the DAGs were further evaluated as potential confounders using the change-in-estimate criterion, whereby a variable was considered a confounder if its inclusion in the model produced a meaningful change ($\geq$10%) in the OR for the association between exposure and outcome. Alcohol and tobacco consumption were assessed using this approach; however, they were not included in the final models, as their inclusion did not yield meaningful changes in the effect estimates. Statistical significance for all logistic models was determined using a p-value threshold of <0.05. All analyses were conducted using Stata Statistical Software, version 19.5 (StataCorp, College Station, TX, USA).

3. Results

The characteristics of nursing students and their differences according to their sleep disturbance and depression status are summarized in Table 1. The participants' ages ranged from 18 to 31 years, with women comprising 80.8% of the total. Most were single, had no children, were unemployed, had a family income of less than $470, were in their second year of university, and did not have a university scholarship. Furthermore, 12.1% of the participants reported consuming alcohol, and 10.2% reported using tobacco at least once per week. In addition, most participants reported spending 3–5 h per day on social media.

Table 1. Sociodemographic, academic, and behavioral characteristics of undergraduate nursing students according to sleep disturbance and depressive symptoms.

Features	Total (n = 638)	Sleep Disturbance			Depression		
		No (n = 308)	Yes (n = 330)	p-Value [a]	No (n = 462)	Yes (n = 176)	p-Value [a]
	f (%)	f (%)	f (%)		f (%)	f (%)	
Sex							
Woman	516 (80.8)	244 (47.3)	272 (52.7)	0.304	380 (73.6)	136 (26.4)	0.153
Man	122 (19.1)	64 (52.5)	58 (47.5)		82 (67.2)	40 (32.8)	
Age							
18–20 years	414 (64.9)	191 (46.1)	223 (53.9)	0.287	290 (70.1)	124 (29.9)	0.138
21–23 years	185 (29.0)	95 (51.4)	90 (48.6)		140 (75.7)	45 (24.3)	
≥24 years	39 (6.1)	22 (56.4)	17 (43.6)		32 (82.1)	7 (17.9)	
Family history of mental illness							
Yes	101 (7.2)	43 (42.6)	58 (57.4)	0.211	57 (56.4)	44 (43.6)	0.001
No	537 (92.8)	265 (49.4)	272 (50.6)		405 (75.4)	132 (24.6)	
Study site							
Durango	280 (43.9)	191 (46.1)	223 (53.9)	0.287	196 (70.0)	84 (30.0)	0.129
Hidalgo	286 (44.8)	95 (51.3)	90 (48.7)		207 (72.4)	79 (27.6)	
Mexico City	72 (11.3)	22 (56.4)	17 (43.6)		59 (81.9)	13 (18.1)	
Marital status							
No partner	601 (94.2)	289 (48.1)	312 (51.9)	0.700	433 (72.1)	168 (27.9)	0.403
With partner	37 (5.8)	19 (51.4)	18 (48.6)		29 (78.4)	8 (21.6)	
Family monthly income							
<470 American dollars	373 (58.6)	169 (45.3)	204 (54.7)	0.075	259 (69.4)	114 (30.6)	0.046
≥470 American dollars	265 (41.5)	139 (52.5)	126 (47.5)		203 (76.6)	62 (23.4)	
Offspring							
Yes	46 (7.2)	13 (28.3)	33 (71.7)	0.005	32 (69.6)	14 (30.4)	0.654
No	592 (92.8)	295 (49.8)	297 (50.2)		430 (72.6)	162 (27.4)	
Year in program							
First	175 (27.4)	84 (48.0)	91 (52.0)	0.550	133 (76.0)	42 (24.0)	0.419
Second	187 (29.3)	94 (50.3)	93 (49.7)		132 (70.6)	55 (29.4)	
Third	164 (25.7)	72 (43.9)	92 (56.1)		113 (68.9)	51 (31.1)	
Fourth	112 (17.6)	58 (51.8)	54 (48.2)		84 (75.0)	28 (25.0)	
Scholarship							
Yes	29 (4.5)	13 (44.8)	16 (55.2)	0.704	18 (62.1)	11 (37.9)	0.202
No	609 (95.5)	295 (48.4)	314 (51.6)		444 (72.9)	165 (27.1)	

Table 1. *Cont.*

Features	Total (n = 638)	Sleep Disturbance No (n = 308)	Sleep Disturbance Yes (n = 330)	*p*-Value [a]	Depression No (n = 462)	Depression Yes (n = 176)	*p*-Value [a]
	f (%)	f (%)	f (%)		f (%)	f (%)	
Employment							
Yes	162 (25.4)	86 (53.1)	76 (46.9)	0.156	40 (24.7)	122 (75.3)	0.340
No	476 (74.6)	222 (46.6)	254 (53.4)		340 (71.4)	136 (28.6)	
Mother's education							
Primary education	76 (11.9)	32 (42.1)	44 (57.9)	0.139	49 (64.5)	24 (35.5)	0.028
Lower secondary education	271 (42.5)	123 (45.4)	148 (54.6)		190 (70.1)	81 (29.9)	
Upper secondary education	195 (30.6)	98 (50.3)	97 (49.7)		144 (73.8)	51 (26.2)	
Tertiary education	96 (15.0)	55 (57.3)	41 (42.7)		80 (83.3)	16 (16.7)	
Father's education							
Primary education	54 (8.5)	26 (48.2)	28 (51.8)	0.849	36 (66.7)	18 (33.3)	0.269
Lower secondary education	271 (42.5)	130 (48.0)	141 (52.0)		189 (69.7)	82 (30.3)	
Upper secondary education	185 (29.0)	86 (46.5)	99 (53.5)		141 (76.2)	44 (23.8)	
Tertiary education	128 (20.0)	66 (51.6)	62 (48.4)		97 (75.8)	31 (24.2)	
Regular alcohol consumption							
Yes	77 (12.1)	45 (58.4)	32 (41.6)	0.057	54 (70.2)	23 (29.8)	0.609
No	561 (87.9)	263 (46.9)	298 (53.1)		409 (72.9)	152 (27.1)	
Regular cigarette smoking							
Yes	65 (10.2)	37 (56.9)	28 (43.1)	0.141	46 (70.7)	19 (29.3)	0.731
No	573 (89.8)	271 (47.3)	302 (52.7)		417 (72.7)	156 (27.3)	
Hours on social media per day							
≤2 h	135 (21.2)	82 (60.7)	53 (39.3)	0.003	112 (52.3)	23 (17.0)	<0.001
3–5 h	287 (45.0)	133 (46.3)	154(53.7)		217 (75.6)	70 (24.4)	
6–8 h	160 (25.0)	74 (46.2)	86(53.8)		104 (65.0)	56 (35.0)	
≥9 h	56 (8.8)	19 (33.9)	37(66.1)		30 (53.6)	26 (46.4)	

Abbreviations: f, frequency. [a] Comparing subjects by sleep disturbance and depression status using Pearson's chi-squared test.

Overall, 51.7% of the participants showed signs of sleep disturbance, and 27.5% showed signs of depression. Among students with sleep disturbances, a higher proportion reported having offspring and spending between three and five hours per day on social media, compared to those with good sleep quality. Similarly, among participants with depression, a greater proportion had lower monthly household income and lower maternal educational attainment, relative to those without depression. Furthermore, the prevalence of depression increased among students who reported spending more time on social media.

The distribution of sleep disturbance and depressive symptoms across levels of problematic social media use is presented in Table 2. The prevalence of sleep problems increased steadily with greater dependence severity, ranging from 36.8% among non-dependent participants to 69.2% among those with high dependence. A similar gradient was observed for depressive symptoms.

After adjusting for potential confounders, students with mild social media dependence showed a higher, but not statistically significant, probability of reporting sleep disturbances compared with non-dependent peers (aOR = 1.31; 95% CI: 0.81–2.10). In contrast, those with moderate (aOR = 2.22; 95% CI: 1.37–3.61) and high dependence (aOR = 3.73; 95% CI: 2.19–6.35) had markedly increased odds of experiencing sleep problems. The magnitude of this association increased progressively across dependence categories, with substantially higher values in the moderate and high groups than in the mild group. Furthermore, a dose–response trend was observed between social media dependence and sleep disturbance (p for trend = 0.001; see Table 3).

Table 2. Sleep disturbance and depressive symptoms by levels of social media addiction.

Social Media Addiction	Total	Sleep Disturbance			Depressive Symptoms		
		No	Yes	*p*-Value [a]	No	Yes	*p*-Value [a]
	f (%)	f (%)	f (%)	f (%)	f (%)	f (%)	f (%)
No addiction	125 (19.6)	79 (63.2)	46 (36.8)	<0.001	104 (83.2)	21 (16.8)	<0.001
Mild dependence	205 (32.1)	115 (56.1)	90 (43.9)		171 (83.4)	34 (16.6)	
Moderate dependence	175 (27.4)	73 (41.7)	102 (58.2)		113(64.6)	62 (35.4)	
High dependency	133 (20.9)	41 (30.8)	92 (69.2)		74 (55.6)	59 (44.4)	

Abbreviations: f, frequency. [a] Comparing subjects by depression and sleep disturbance status using Pearson's chi-squared test.

Table 3. Raw and adjusted odds ratios of the relationship between problematic social media use and sleep disturbance.

Problematic Social Media Use	Sleep Disturbance			
	OR (95% IC)	*p*-Value	OR [a] (95% CI)	*p*-Value
No addiction	Ref.		Ref.	
Mild dependence	1.34 (0.85, 2.12)	0.204	1.31 (0.81, 2.10)	0.263
Moderate dependence	2.39 (1.49, 3.84)	<0.001	2.22 (1.37, 3.61)	0.001
High dependency	3.85 (2.29, 6.49)	<0.001	3.73 (2.19, 6.35)	<0.001
p-trend	<0.001		<0.001	

Abbreviations: OR, odds ratio; CI, Confidence interval. [a] Adjusted for age, sex, year in program, paid work, family monthly income, study location, family history of mental illness, and parental education.

No statistically significant association was found between mild social media dependence and depressive symptoms. In contrast, students with moderate (aOR = 2.56; 95% CI: 1.41–4.64) and high dependence (aOR = 4.54; 95% CI: 2.45–8.44) showed a significantly greater likelihood of presenting depressive symptoms compared with those without problematic social media use. The magnitude of this association increased progressively across dependence categories, and a clear dose–response trend was observed between social media use and depressive symptomatology (p for trend < 0.001; see Table 4).

Table 4. Raw and adjusted odds ratios of the relationship between problematic social media use and depressive symptoms.

Problematic Social Media Use	Depressive Symptoms			
	OR (95% CI)	*p*-Value	OR [a] (95% CI)	*p*-Value
No addiction	Ref.		Ref.	
Mild dependence	0.98 (0.54, 1.78)	0.960	1.05 (0.63, 2.09)	0.872
Moderate dependence	2.71 (1.54, 4.76)	<0.001	2.56 (1.41, 4.64)	0.002
High dependency	3.94 (2.20, 7.05)	<0.001	4.54 (2.45, 8.44)	<0.001
	<0.001		<0.001	

Abbreviations: OR, odds ratio; CI, Confidence interval. [a] Adjusted for age, sex, year in program, paid work, family monthly income, study location, family history of mental illness, and parental education.

Figure 1 summarizes the results of the mediation analysis. Our findings indicate that the association between problematic social media use and depressive symptoms was partially mediated by sleep disturbance, which accounted for 31.4% of the total effect. The indirect pathway was statistically significant (adjusted odds ratio [aOR] = 1.22; 95% confidence interval [CI] = 1.01, 1.38), while the direct effect remained substantial (aOR = 1.57; 95% CI = 1.03, 2.39). These results suggest that, although sleep disturbance plays a mediating role, most of the association (68.6%) is likely explained by other mechanisms.

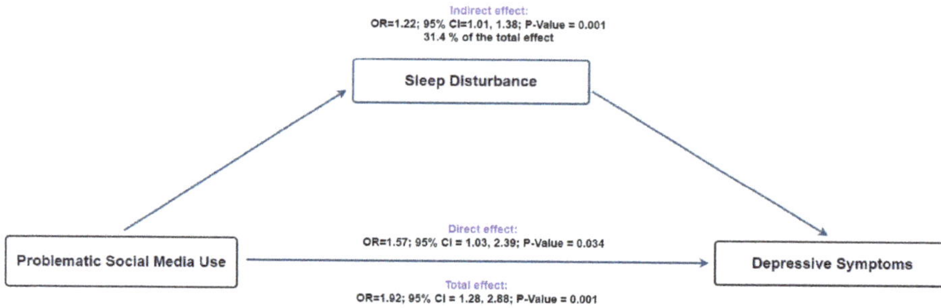

Figure 1. Counterfactual mediation model of problematic social media use, sleep disturbance, and depressive symptoms.

To evaluate the robustness of these findings, a sensitivity analysis was performed using an alternative definition of problematic social media use. In this model, participants with no or mild addiction were grouped as a single reference category, and those with moderate or severe addiction were classified as having problematic use. The mediation analysis under this dichotomized classification yielded a natural indirect effect of 1.21 (95% CI 1.07–1.36; *p*-value = 0.002) and a natural direct effect of 2.41 (95% CI 1.69–3.43; *p*-value = 0.001). The proportion mediated through sleep disturbance was 20% (95% CI 0.06–0.33). The consistency of these estimates with those of the main model supports the stability of the observed relationships (Supplementary Figure S2).

4. Discussion

Our findings revealed a significant association between problematic social media use and depressive symptoms, with sleep disturbances accounting for a modest but statistically significant proportion of this relationship.

In our study, 51.7% of participants reported poor sleep quality, a substantial proportion, though notably lower than the 80% prevalence reported in a recent study from Tamaulipas, Mexico, despite both using the same measurement tool (Pérez et al., 2024). This discrepancy may be explained by methodological differences, such as the smaller sample size in the previous study (n = 99), as well as by contextual and academic differences across institutions. Additionally, the limited set of covariates considered in that study may have restricted the exploration of other relevant psychosocial factors. In contrast, our multicenter design, spanning different regions of the country, provides a more comprehensive and representative perspective.

Moreover, compared with findings from the international literature, the prevalence of sleep disturbance observed in our study falls within the expected range, typically reported as 30–50% in similar student populations (Efstathiou et al., 2025; Ibrahim et al., 2024). This consistency supports the robustness of our estimates and reinforces the relevance of sleep disturbance as a common concern in this demographic group.

In our study, the prevalence of depressive symptoms was 27.5%. This estimate contrasts with findings from two recent studies conducted in Mexico. Márquez-Ríos and Grimaldo-Zapata (2024) reported a prevalence of 15.5%, whereas Bueno-Brito et al. (2024) documented a markedly higher prevalence of 52.36%. These discrepancies could be attributed to various methodological differences, such as the instrument used to assess depression and the smaller sample size, both of which were smaller than in our study. Furthermore, in the Bueno-Brito et al. (2024) study, the sample consisted exclusively of first-year students. The transition to university life represents a particularly challenging period, characterized by separation from family life, increased academic demands, and the need to assume new personal and professional responsibilities. These factors, combined, make the first year of university a particularly vulnerable time for mental health.

In the international context, a systematic review with meta-analysis reported an overall prevalence of depression of 29% in nursing students (Efstathiou et al., 2025), a figure closer to that observed in our study. However, it is essential to note that a few of the primary studies included in this meta-analysis were conducted in Latin American students; thus, the prevalence of this affective problem in the region may not be adequately represented. Despite this, the figures above reaffirm that depression constitutes a significant mental health problem among nursing students around the world.

Our findings showed that moderate and high levels of social media dependence were associated with a greater likelihood of sleep disturbance. The association followed a clear gradient, with higher dependence levels corresponding to increasingly frequent sleep problems, supporting a dose–response relationship between social media use and sleep quality. Our findings are consistent with several previous studies conducted in nursing students and the general university population, which have documented that addictive use of social media and smartphones is associated with altered sleep patterns (Haddaouy et al., 2025; Kalal et al., 2023; Rahman et al., 2025; Setyowati et al., 2023; Zhu et al., 2023).

Several underlying mechanisms could explain the observed association. During the night, in the absence of sunlight, the retina sends signals to the suprachiasmatic nucleus of the hypothalamus (considered the body's biological clock), which stimulates the pineal gland to produce and release melatonin into the blood. This hormone primarily regulates the circadian rhythm, especially the sleep–wake cycle (Patel et al., 2025; Pevet et al., 2021). Nevertheless, exposure to artificial light, including that emitted by electronic devices such as tablets, computers, and mobile phones (commonly used for checking social media), can mimic natural sunlight, interfering with melatonin synthesis and consequently disrupting standard sleep patterns (Allen et al., 2018; Blume et al., 2019; Kumar et al., 2025). Likewise, constant interaction with social media, especially at night, can lead to cognitive activation, making it difficult to fall asleep and reducing its quality (Firth et al., 2019; Joshi, 2022). Furthermore, the highly stimulating or entertaining content often found on these platforms can increase alertness and prolong vigilance. On the other hand, stressful content, social comparison, and the pressure to stay connected can also generate anxiety or emotional distress, which in turn contributes to a greater vulnerability to sleep disorders (O. Ahmed et al., 2024; Korte, 2020).

Consistent with the previously described associations, we found that problematic social media use is significantly associated with higher odds of having depressive symptoms. This finding is consistent with reports from different studies, which have documented that problematic use of these platforms is linked to a negative impact on the mental health of nursing students and generally young people (Cai et al., 2021; David et al., 2024; Jiayuan et al., 2025; Osman, 2025).

In this context, compulsive social media use can interfere with daily routines, affect motivation for activities outside the digital environment, lead to difficulties in setting personal boundaries, and result in feelings of frustration, all of which contribute to a deterioration in emotional well-being (M. Ahmed, 2023; Firth et al., 2024). The intermittent feedback provided by these platforms (based on notifications, social interactions, and virtual rewards) could reinforce addictive behaviors and fuel negative emotional states when expectations are not met. This pattern of interaction can generate a vicious cycle in which excessive social media use becomes both a cause and a consequence of depression (J. Wang & Wang, 2025).

It is important to note that, in our analysis, mild social media dependence was not significantly associated with either depression or sleep disturbances. This may reflect frequent but non-dysfunctional use, which is common and often adaptive among university students, given the academic and social utility of these platforms. From a methodological standpoint, the instrument's sensitivity to detect subtle impairments may be limited, and its classification thresholds may not clearly distinguish between intensive but functional use and early signs of problematic behavior. Additionally, the sample size within this category might have been insufficient to detect modest associations. Nonetheless, the significant trend across dependence levels supports a dose–response pattern, indicating that the adverse effects of social media use increase progressively with greater dependence intensity (Abi-Jaoude et al., 2020; Geng & Liu, 2025; Soraci et al., 2024; Yan et al., 2024).

Through our mediation analysis, we identified that sleep disturbances partially mediated the overall effect of problematic social media use on depressive symptoms. Specifically, a significant indirect effect through these disturbances was found, explaining approximately 31.4% of the total association.

This finding underscores the potential role of sleep disturbance as a biological and behavioral pathway linking problematic social media use to depression. Sleep disturbances can directly affect the neuroendocrine, immune systems, and neurotransmitter systems, all of which are implicated in the pathophysiology of depression. Partial or chronic sleep deprivation can disrupt the hypothalamic–pituitary–adrenal (HPA) axis, leading to increased cortisol secretion, a hormone closely associated with stress and depression (Dziurkowska & Wesolowski, 2021; Nicolaides et al., 2000). Sleep disruption is also linked to reduced availability of serotonin and dopamine (Moncrieff et al., 2023). Moreover, sleep fragmentation and decreased deep sleep have been linked to increased systemic inflammation, as reflected in elevated markers such as interleukin-6 (IL-6) and C-reactive protein, which have also been implicated in the etiology of depression (Nishuty et al., 2019).

On the other hand, sleep disorders have the potential to weaken a person's coping strategies when dealing with daily stress (Palmer & Alfano, 2017). Lack of adequate rest impairs emotional self-regulation, which increases people's vulnerability to experiencing intense negative emotions, such as depression, in the face of stressful events (Y. Wang et al., 2023). This may be especially relevant in the university context, where students face multiple academic, social, and personal pressures. In this sense, a lack of sleep could play a modulating role, amplifying the negative emotional impact of inappropriate social media use.

Although sleep disturbances partially mediated the relationship, explaining 31.4% of the total effect, a substantial proportion (68.6%) remains unexplained, suggesting the presence of additional mechanisms that should be explored in future studies. Previous evidence has identified several potential pathways, including increased exposure to social comparison and idealized content, which could negatively impact self-esteem and mood (Samra et al., 2022). Additionally, experiences such as online harassment or exposure to distressing content may contribute to depression independently of sleep (Alghamdi et al., 2025; Ye & Gao, 2025). Excessive social media use may also lead to social withdrawal or reduced face-to-face interaction, fostering feelings of isolation. Finally, maladaptive emotional regulation strategies, such as using social media to escape from negative emotions, may reinforce depressive symptoms over time. These alternative pathways warrant further investigation in future studies using comprehensive models that integrate psychological, behavioral, and contextual factors.

In addition to these behavioral and cognitive mechanisms, the partial mediation observed could also reflect a conceptual overlap between sleep disturbances and depressive symptomatology. Difficulty initiating or maintaining sleep is not only a diagnostic criterion for depression but also a factor that functionally disrupts emotion regulation, increases cognitive rumination, and heightens stress reactivity (Jansson-Fröjmark & Hossain, 2024; W. Wang et al., 2024). These psychological processes can amplify negative mood and reduce resilience to daily stressors, thereby reinforcing the depressive pathway. Importantly, in our study, sleep quality and depression were assessed using independent, validated instruments that capture distinct but interconnected domains (Pace-Schott et al., 2023). Therefore, the mediating effect of sleep disturbances likely represents both shared pathophysiological mechanisms and functional psychological processes through which inadequate sleep contributes to the onset and persistence of depressive symptoms.

To verify the stability of these findings, a sensitivity analysis was conducted using an alternative definition of social media addiction, in which the categories none and mild addiction were combined and compared with moderate and severe addiction. The results remained consistent with those of the main model, confirming that sleep disturbance continued to play a mediating role in the relationship between social media addiction and depressive symptoms. However, the proportion of the total effect explained through this pathway was smaller, which may reflect the greater predominance of direct mechanisms among individuals with more severe levels of social media use. These results support the robustness of our findings and highlight the complexity of the pathways linking problematic social media use to mental health outcomes.

Limitations and Strengths

This study has some limitations that should be acknowledged. First, the cross-sectional design of our study does not allow for establishing a temporal sequence between social media addiction and sleep disturbances or depressive symptoms; therefore, the associations we estimate are not causal and should be interpreted with caution. Second, the variables were assessed using questionnaires; thus, participants' data on social media use, sleep quality, or depressive symptoms could have been underestimated or overestimated. Furthermore, although validated instruments were used, they assess perceived symptoms or behaviors and do not replace clinical diagnostic evaluations. Nevertheless, this approach is common in epidemiological studies. Third, although the study included participants from three public universities in different Mexican states, which enhances representativeness within nursing programs, the findings may not be generalizable to students in private institutions, other academic disciplines, or other cultural contexts. However, the associations identified in this study are consistent with well-established biological mechanisms that link excessive screen exposure with sleep disturbance and depression. These mechanisms are not culturally bound, which supports the potential external validity of our findings beyond the studied population.

Despite the limitations above, this study has significant strengths. It is one of the first multicenter studies in Mexico to jointly analyze social media addiction, sleep quality, and depressive symptoms in nursing students, a population particularly vulnerable to academic, social, and emotional stressors. Since validated tests were used in the Mexican population and were administered by trained personnel, it is unlikely that our findings were affected by differential misclassification bias.

Additionally, the sample size was large and statistically justified, and the stratified sampling method adequately represented students from three public institutions in different regions of the country. Finally, the statistical models were adjusted for confounding variables, using DAGs and statistical criteria for identification, enhancing the robustness and internal validity of the findings.

5. Conclusions

Problematic social media use was associated with depressive symptoms among Mexican undergraduate nursing students, and the findings suggest that sleep disturbances may partially mediate this relationship. Our results highlight the importance of addressing problematic social media use as an emerging psychosocial risk factor in the university setting. They underscore the importance of implementing preventive strategies in academic nursing programs that foster healthy, critical use of digital technologies, promote balanced digital habits, and actively safeguard students' mental health.

From a practical perspective, these findings pave the way for educational interventions, workshops, and institutional policies that integrate digital literacy, emotional self-care, and sleep hygiene as essential components of nursing staff training. Furthermore, the results can guide the design of psychoeducational support programs that identify and address risky digital behaviors and their consequences early. At the institutional level, nursing schools must recognize the impact of the digital environment on mental health and develop comprehensive student wellness policies that address the academic, technological, and psycho-emotional factors influencing professional performance during training.

While the mechanisms linking social media use, sleep disturbance, and depression are biologically universal, their contextual expression may differ across educational and cultural settings. By confirming this mediational pattern among Mexican nursing students using a counterfactual framework, our findings strengthen the external validity of previous evidence and highlight the need for culturally responsive strategies to promote mental well-being among healthcare students.

Supplementary Materials: The following supporting information can be downloaded at: https://www.mdpi.com/article/10.3390/ejihpe15110229/s1, Supplementary Table S1. Distribution of the Study Sample by Recruitment Site Based on Proportional Stratified Sampling; Supplementary Figure S1: Directed acyclic graph for the hypothesized counterfactual mediation structure in which social media addiction influences depressive symptoms directly and indirectly through sleep disturbance; Supplementary Figure S2: Sensitivity analysis of the mediation model.

Author Contributions: Conceptualization, J.Á.H.-M., A.C.C.-M. and M.A.C.-D.; methodology, J.Á.H.-M. and A.C.C.-M.; software, J.Á.H.-M. and A.C.C.-M.; validation, M.A.C.-D., G.M.O.-R., R.C.-D., F.V.-R., Y.C.O.-O., M.T.-M. and E.A.C.-E.; formal analysis, J.Á.H.-M. and A.C.C.-M.; investigation, J.Á.H.-M., G.M.O.-R., R.C.-D., F.V.-R., E.A.C.-E. and A.C.C.-M.; resources, M.A.C.-D.; data curation, J.Á.H.-M., A.C.C.-M. and Y.C.O.-O.; writing—original draft preparation, J.Á.H.-M. and A.C.C.-M.; writing—review and editing, M.A.C.-D., G.M.O.-R., R.C.-D., F.V.-R., Y.C.O.-O., M.T.-M. and E.A.C.-E.; visualization, J.Á.H.-M., G.M.O.-R., R.C.-D., F.V.-R., E.A.C.-E., Y.C.O.-O., M.T.-M. and A.C.C.-M.; supervision, M.A.C.-D.; project administration, M.A.C.-D. All authors have read and agreed to the published version of the manuscript.

Funding: This research received no external funding.

Institutional Review Board Statement: The study was conducted in accordance with the Declaration of Helsinki, and approved by Hospital Juarez of Mexico's Ethics and Research Committee (protocol code HJM-036-23I, approve date 31 October 2023).

Informed Consent Statement: Informed consent was obtained from all subjects involved in this study.

Data Availability Statement: The data that support the findings of this study are openly available in Mendeley Data at doi: 10.17632/y478b26pnc.1; https://data.mendeley.com/datasets/y478b26pnc/1 (accessed on 11 August 2025).

Conflicts of Interest: The authors declare no conflicts of interest.

Abbreviations

The following abbreviations are used in this manuscript:

CESD-7	Center for Epidemiologic Studies Depression Scale
SMAS-SF	Social Media Addiction Scale-Student Form

PSQI	Pittsburgh Sleep Quality Index
OR	Odds ratio
CI	Confidence interval
DAGs	Directed acyclic graphs

References

Abi-Jaoude, E., Naylor, K. T., & Pignatiello, A. (2020). Smartphones, social media use and youth mental health. *CMAJ: Canadian Medical Association Journal*, *192*(6), E136–E141. [CrossRef]

Ahmed, M. (2023). Psychological impact of social media addiction on interpersonal relationships in Pakistan. *International Journal of Psychology*, *8*(4), 53–64. [CrossRef]

Ahmed, O., Walsh, E. I., Dawel, A., Alateeq, K., Espinoza Oyarce, D. A., & Cherbuin, N. (2024). Social media use, mental health and sleep: A systematic review with meta-analyses. *Journal of Affective Disorders*, *367*, 701–712. [CrossRef]

Akhtar, P., Ma, L., Waqas, A., Naveed, S., Li, Y., Rahman, A., & Wang, Y. (2020). Prevalence of depression among university students in low and middle income countries (LMICs): A systematic review and meta-analysis. *Journal of Affective Disorders*, *274*, 911–919. [CrossRef] [PubMed]

AlAmer, M., Shdaifat, E., Alshowkan, A., Eldeen, A. G., & Jamama, A. (2020). Exploring associations between internet addiction, depressive symptoms, and sleep disturbance among saudi nursing students. *The Open Nursing Journal*, *14*(1), 14–29. [CrossRef]

Alghamdi, W., Almadani, S., Banjer, H., Alsulami, D., & Alghamdi, Y. (2025). Relationship between cyberbullying, anxiety, and depression among university students in Jeddah, Saudi Arabia: A cross-sectional study. *International Journal of Psychiatry in Medicine*, *60*(2), 170–186. [CrossRef] [PubMed]

Alimoradi, Z., Lin, C.-Y., Broström, A., Bülow, P. H., Bajalan, Z., Griffiths, M. D., Ohayon, M. M., & Pakpour, A. H. (2019). Internet addiction and sleep problems: A systematic review and meta-analysis. *Sleep Medicine Reviews*, *47*, 51–61. [CrossRef]

Allen, A. E., Hazelhoff, E. M., Martial, F. P., Cajochen, C., & Lucas, R. J. (2018). Exploiting metamerism to regulate the impact of a visual display on alertness and melatonin suppression independent of visual appearance. *Sleep*, *41*(8), zsy100. [CrossRef] [PubMed]

Alonzo, R., Hussain, J., Stranges, S., & Anderson, K. K. (2021). Interplay between social media use, sleep quality, and mental health in youth: A systematic review. *Sleep Medicine Reviews*, *56*, 101414. [CrossRef]

Amirthalingam, J., & Khera, A. (2024). Understanding social media addiction: A deep dive. *Cureus*, *16*(10), e72499. [CrossRef]

Berdida, D. J. E. (2025). Nursing students' personality traits, sleep quality, social media addiction, and academic performance: A multi-site structural equation model analysis. *Journal of Professional Nursing*, *56*, 26–35. [CrossRef]

Blume, C., Garbazza, C., & Spitschan, M. (2019). Effects of light on human circadian rhythms, sleep and mood. *Somnologie*, *23*(3), 147–156. [CrossRef]

Bueno-Brito, C., Pérez-Castro, E., & Delgado-Delgado, J. (2024). Adicción a teléfonos inteligentes, ansiedad, depresión y estrés en estudiantes de enfermería mexicanos. *Revista Cuidarte*, *15*(3), e3814. [CrossRef]

Byeon, S., & Lee, W. (2023). An introduction to causal mediation analysis with a comparison of 2 R packages. *Journal of Preventive Medicine and Public Health = Yebang Uihakhoe Chi*, *56*(4), 303–311. [CrossRef] [PubMed]

Cai, H., Xi, H.-T., An, F., Wang, Z., Han, L., Liu, S., Zhu, Q., Bai, W., Zhao, Y.-J., Chen, L., Ge, Z.-M., Ji, M., Zhang, H., Yang, B.-X., Chen, P., Cheung, T., Jackson, T., Tang, Y.-L., & Xiang, Y.-T. (2021). The association between internet addiction and anxiety in nursing students: A network analysis. *Frontiers in Psychiatry*, *12*, 723355. [CrossRef]

Cañón-Montañez, W., & Rodríguez-Acelas, A. (2019). Use of Causal Diagrams for Nursing Research: A tool for application in epidemiological studies—PMC. *Investigación y Educación en Enfermería*, *37*(1), e01. [CrossRef] [PubMed]

Carmona-Huerta, J., Durand-Arias, S., Rodriguez, A., Guarner-Catalá, C., Cardona-Muller, D., Madrigal-de-León, E., & Alvarado, R. (2021). Community mental health care in Mexico: A regional perspective from a mid-income country. *International Journal of Mental Health Systems*, *15*(1), 7. [CrossRef]

Consuelos-Sánchez, K. S., Cano-Estrada, A., Castañeda-Márquez, A. C., & Hernández-Mariano, J. Á. (2023). Nursing training and its association with burnout syndrome among Mexican undergraduate students. *Salud Mental*, *46*(2), 97–104. [CrossRef]

Corke, L., Maksyutynska, K., Jones, J. M., & George, T. P. (2025). The relationship between social media use, and mental health disorders in adolescents and young adults: A scoping review. *Annals of Clinical Psychiatry*, *36*(3), 89–99. [CrossRef]

Cvetković-Vega, A., Maguiña, J. L., Soto, A., Lama-Valdivia, J., & López, L. E. C. (2021). Cross-sectional studies. *Revista de la Facultad de Medicina Humana*, *21*(1), 179–185. [CrossRef]

David, L., Ismaiel, A., Foucambert, P., Leucuta, D. C., Popa, S.-L., Fadgyas Stanculete, M., & Dumitrascu, D. L. (2024). Mental disorders, social media addiction, and academic performance in Romanian undergraduate nursing students. *Journal of Clinical Medicine*, *13*(15), 4475. [CrossRef] [PubMed]

Digitale, J. C., Martin, J. N., & Glymour, M. M. (2022). Tutorial on directed acyclic graphs. *Journal of Clinical Epidemiology*, *142*, 264–267. [CrossRef] [PubMed]

Dresp-Langley, B., & Hutt, A. (2022). Digital addiction and sleep. *International Journal of Environmental Research and Public Health*, *19*(11), 6910. [CrossRef] [PubMed]

Dziurkowska, E., & Wesolowski, M. (2021). Cortisol as a biomarker of mental disorder severity. *Journal of Clinical Medicine*, *10*(21), 5204. [CrossRef]

Efstathiou, M., Kakaidi, V., Tsitsas, G., Mantzoukas, S., Gouva, M., & Dragioti, E. (2025). The prevalence of mental health issues among nursing students: An umbrella review synthesis of meta-analytic evidence. *International Journal of Nursing Studies*, *163*, 104993. [CrossRef]

Fan, Y., Fan, A., Yang, Z., & Fan, D. (2025). Global burden of mental disorders in 204 countries and territories, 1990–2021: Results from the global burden of disease study 2021. *BMC Psychiatry*, *25*(1), 486. [CrossRef]

Firth, J., Torous, J., López-Gil, J. F., Linardon, J., Milton, A., Lambert, J., Smith, L., Jarić, I., Fabian, H., Vancampfort, D., Onyeaka, H., Schuch, F. B., & Firth, J. A. (2024). From "online brains" to "online lives": Understanding the individualized impacts of Internet use across psychological, cognitive and social dimensions. *World Psychiatry*, *23*(2), 176–190. [CrossRef]

Firth, J., Torous, J., Stubbs, B., Firth, J. A., Steiner, G. Z., Smith, L., Alvarez-Jimenez, M., Gleeson, J., Vancampfort, D., Armitage, C. J., & Sarris, J. (2019). The "online brain": How the Internet may be changing our cognition. *World Psychiatry*, *18*(2), 119–129. [CrossRef]

Geng, Z., & Liu, R. (2025). The impact of smartphone addiction and negative emotions on parent–child relationships among elementary school students. *Frontiers in Psychiatry*, *16*, 1582741. [CrossRef]

Haddaouy, A. E., Miyah, Y., Benjelloun, M., Mengad, A., Blaak, H., Iziki, H., & Omari, F. E. (2025). Smartphone addiction and sleep quality among nursing students in Meknes, Morocco: A cross-sectional study. *Belitung Nursing Journal*, *11*(2), 133–141. [CrossRef]

Hernández-Mariano, J. Á., Hurtado-Salgado, E., Velázquez-Núñez, M. D. C., & Cupul-Uicab, L. A. (2024). Prevalence of academic burnout among nursing students: A systematic review and meta-analysis. *Journal of Nursing Education*, *63*(8), 533–539. [CrossRef]

Hicks, R., & Tingley, D. (2011). Causal mediation analysis. *The Stata Journal*, *11*(4), 605–619. [CrossRef]

Ibrahim, F. M., Salmi, R. N., Saif, M. A., & Mohammed, A. (2024). Sleep disorders' prevalence and impact on academic performance among undergraduate nursing students in a selected university, United Arab Emirates. *SAGE Open Nursing*, *10*, 23779608241274229. [CrossRef]

Jansson-Fröjmark, M., & Hossain, S. (2024). Emotion dysregulation in insomnia disorder: The possible role of psychiatric comorbidity. *Frontiers in Sleep*, *3*, 1383552. [CrossRef]

Jiayuan, Z., Lina, M., & Yang, L. (2025). Problematic media use, mental health literacy, and their interaction in depression among nursing students. *BMC Nursing*, *24*, 199. [CrossRef] [PubMed]

Joshi, S. C. (2022). Sleep latency and sleep disturbances mediates the association between nighttime cell phone use and psychological well-being in college students. *Sleep and Biological Rhythms*, *20*(3), 431–443. [CrossRef] [PubMed]

Jung, S. J. (2021). Introduction to mediation analysis and examples of its application to real-world data. *Journal of Preventive Medicine and Public Health*, *54*(3), 166–172. [CrossRef] [PubMed]

Kalal, N., Vel, N. S., Angmo, S., Choyal, S., Bishnoi, S., Dhaka, S., Rulaniya, S., & Banswal, S. (2023). Smartphone addiction and its impact on quality of sleep and academic performance among nursing students. Institutional based cross-sectional study in Western Rajasthan (India). *Investigación y Educación En Enfermería*, *41*(2), e11. Available online: https://www.redalyc.org/journal/1052/105275612011/html/ (accessed on 29 July 2025). [CrossRef]

Karna, B., Sankari, A., & Tatikonda, G. (2025). Sleep disorder. In *StatPearls*. StatPearls Publishing. Available online: http://www.ncbi.nlm.nih.gov/books/NBK560720/ (accessed on 29 July 2025).

Kinsella, J. E., & Chin, B. N. (2024). Mechanisms linking social media use and sleep in emerging adults in the United States. *Behavioral Sciences*, *14*(9), 794. [CrossRef]

Korte, M. (2020). The impact of the digital revolution on human brain and behavior: Where do we stand? *Dialogues in Clinical Neuroscience*, *22*(2), 101–111. [CrossRef]

Kumar, M., Katoch, O. R., Kumar, N., & Sehgal, S. (2025). Exploring the link between smartphone use and sleep quality: A systematic review. *Sleep Research*, *2*(1), 42–56. [CrossRef]

Labrague, L. J., McEnroe-Petitte, D. M., De Los Santos, J. A. A., & Edet, O. B. (2018). Examining stress perceptions and coping strategies among Saudi nursing students: A systematic review. *Nurse Education Today*, *65*, 192–200. [CrossRef]

Levenson, J. C., Shensa, A., Sidani, J. E., Colditz, J. B., & Primack, B. A. (2017). Social media use before bed and sleep disturbance among young adults in the United States: A nationally representative study. *Sleep*, *40*(9), zsx113. [CrossRef]

Lițan, D.-E. (2025). Online captive: The impact of social media addiction on depression and anxiety—An SEM approach to the mediating role of self-esteem and the moderating effects of age and professional status. *Behavioral Sciences*, *15*(4), 481. [CrossRef]

Liu, Z., Xie, Y., Sun, Z., Liu, D., Yin, H., & Shi, L. (2023). Factors associated with academic burnout and its prevalence among university students: A cross-sectional study. *BMC Medical Education*, *23*(1), 317. [CrossRef] [PubMed]

Márquez-Ríos, M. M. G., & Grimaldo-Zapata, I. P. (2024). Niveles de estrés, ansiedad y depresión en estudiantes de enfermería: Un estudio transversal. *Cuidado Multidisciplinario de la Salud BUAP, 5*(10), 8–20.

Mofatteh, M. (2020). Risk factors associated with stress, anxiety, and depression among university undergraduate students. *AIMS Public Health, 8*(1), 36–65. [CrossRef]

Moncrieff, J., Cooper, R. E., Stockmann, T., Amendola, S., Hengartner, M. P., & Horowitz, M. A. (2023). The serotonin theory of depression: A systematic umbrella review of the evidence. *Molecular Psychiatry, 28*(8), 3243–3256. [CrossRef] [PubMed]

Nicolaides, N. C., Vgontzas, A. N., Kritikou, I., & Chrousos, G. (2000). HPA Axis and Sleep. In K. R. Feingold, S. F. Ahmed, B. Anawalt, M. R. Blackman, A. Boyce, G. Chrousos, E. Corpas, W. W. de Herder, K. Dhatariya, K. Dungan, J. Hofland, S. Kalra, G. Kaltsas, N. Kapoor, C. Koch, P. Kopp, M. Korbonits, C. S. Kovacs, W. Kuohung, ... D. P. Wilson (Eds.), *Endotext*. MDText.com, Inc. Available online: http://www.ncbi.nlm.nih.gov/books/NBK279071/ (accessed on 5 August 2025).

Nishuty, N. L., Khandoker, M. M. H., Karmoker, J. R., Ferdous, S., Shahriar, M., Qusar, M. M. A. S., Islam, M. S., Kadir, M. F., & Islam, M. R. (2019). Evaluation of Serum Interleukin-6 and C-reactive Protein Levels in Drug-naïve Major Depressive Disorder Patients. *Cureus, 11*(1), e3868. [CrossRef]

Ojeda-Paredes, P., Estrella-Castillo, D. F., Rubio-Zapata, H. A., Ojeda-Paredes, P., Estrella-Castillo, D. F., & Rubio-Zapata, H. A. (2019). Sleep quality, insomnia symptoms and academic performance on medicine students. *Investigación En Educación Médica, 8*(29), 36–44. [CrossRef]

Osman, W. A. (2025). Social media use and associated mental health indicators among University students: A cross-sectional study. *Scientific Reports, 15*, 9534. [CrossRef]

Pace-Schott, E. F., Kleim, B., & Alfano, C. A. (2023). Editorial: How does sleep help regulate negative emotion? *Frontiers in Behavioral Neuroscience, 16*, 1125841. [CrossRef] [PubMed]

Palmer, C. A., & Alfano, C. A. (2017). Sleep and emotion regulation: An organizing, integrative review. *Sleep Medicine Reviews, 31*, 6–16. [CrossRef] [PubMed]

Pan American Health Organization. (2025). *Health workforce in the Americas: Data and regional indicators* [La fuerza de trabajo en salud en las Américas: Datos e indicadores regionales]. Available online: https://www.paho.org/es/documentos/fuerza-trabajo-salud-americas-datos-e-indicadores-regionales (accessed on 25 October 2025).

Patel, A. K., Reddy, V., Shumway, K. R., & Araujo, J. F. (2025). Physiology, sleep stages. In *StatPearls*. StatPearls Publishing. Available online: http://www.ncbi.nlm.nih.gov/books/NBK526132/ (accessed on 25 October 2025).

Patino, C. M., & Ferreira, J. C. (2016). Test for trend: Evaluating dose-response effects in association studies. *Jornal Brasileiro de Pneumologia, 42*(4), 240. [CrossRef] [PubMed]

Pevet, P., Challet, E., & Felder-Schmittbuhl, M.-P. (2021). Melatonin and the circadian system: Keys for health with a focus on sleep. *Handbook of Clinical Neurology, 179*, 331–343. [CrossRef]

Pérez, R. L., Flores, D. S. C., Rosas, L. R., Hernández, K. B., Cabrera, B. M., & Gómez, T. G. (2024). Calidad de sueño en estudiantes de la Licenciatura en Enfermería General [Sleep quality among undergraduate nursing students]. *Ciencia Latina Revista Científica Multidisciplinar, 8*(2), 2809–2824. [CrossRef]

Rahman, M., Rabby, M. F., Kabir, M. R., Anjum, R., Saha, O., Bhuiyan, M. A. A., Emon, H. H., & Hossain, M. M. (2025). Associations between social media addiction, social media fatigue, fear of missing out, and sleep quality among university students in Bangladesh: A cross-sectional study. *Journal of Health, Population, and Nutrition, 44*(1), 152. [CrossRef]

Rijnhart, J. J. M., Valente, M. J., Smyth, H. L., & MacKinnon, D. P. (2023). Statistical mediation analysis for models with a binary mediator and a binary outcome: The differences between causal and traditional mediation analysis. *Prevention Science: The Official Journal of the Society for Prevention Research, 24*(3), 408–418. [CrossRef]

Rudman, A., & Gustavsson, J. P. (2012). Burnout during nursing education predicts lower occupational preparedness and future clinical performance: A longitudinal study. *International Journal of Nursing Studies, 49*(8), 988–1001. [CrossRef]

Sahin, C. (2018). Social media addiction scale-student form: The reliability and validity study. *Turkish Online Journal of Educational Technology—TOJET, 17*(1), 169–182.

Salari, N., Zarei, H., Hosseinian-Far, A., Rasoulpoor, S., Shohaimi, S., & Mohammadi, M. (2025). The global prevalence of social media addiction among university students: A systematic review and meta-analysis. *Journal of Public Health, 33*(1), 223–236. [CrossRef]

Salinas-Rodríguez, A., Manrique-Espinoza, B., Acosta-Castillo, G. I., Franco-Núñez, A., Rosas-Carrasco, Ó., Gutiérrez-Robledo, L. M., & Sosa-Ortiz, A. L. (2014). Validación de un punto de corte para la versión breve de la Escala de Depresión del Centro de Estudios Epidemiológicos en adultos mayores mexicanos [Validation of a cutoff point for the short version of the Center for Epidemiologic Studies Depression Scale in Mexican older adults]. *Salud Pública de México, 56*(3), 279–285.

Samra, A., Warburton, W. A., & Collins, A. M. (2022). Social comparisons: A potential mechanism linking problematic social media use with depression. *Journal of Behavioral Addictions, 11*(2), 607–614. [CrossRef]

Scott, A. J., Webb, T. L., Martyn-St James, M., Rowse, G., & Weich, S. (2021). Improving sleep quality leads to better mental health: A meta-analysis of randomised controlled trials. *Sleep Medicine Reviews, 60*, 101556. [CrossRef]

Setyowati, L., Kurnia, A. D., Lestari, W., & Karuncharernpanit, S. (2023). Association between social media addiction and sleep quality among undergraduate nursing students: A cross-sectional study. *Frontiers of Nursing*, *10*(2), 233–239. [CrossRef]

Silva, V., Chiquito, N. C., Andrade, R. A. P. O., Brito, M. F. P., & Camelo, S. H. H. (2011). Fatores de estresse no último ano do curso de graduação em enfermagem: Percepção dos estudantes [Stress factors in the final year of undergraduate nursing education: Students' perception]. *Revista Enfermagem UERJ*, *19*(1), 121–126.

Sonmez, Y., Akdemir, M., Meydanlioglu, A., & Aktekin, M. R. (2023). Psychological distress, depression, and anxiety in nursing students: A longitudinal study. *Healthcare*, *11*(5), 636. [CrossRef] [PubMed]

Soraci, P., Pisanti, R., Servidio, R., Holte, A. J., Ferrari, A., Demetrovics, Z., & Griffiths, M. D. (2024). The associations between the problematic social media and smartphone use, social phobia, and self-esteem: A structural equation modeling analysis. *International Journal of Mental Health and Addiction*. [CrossRef]

Tennant, P. W. G., Murray, E. J., Arnold, K. F., Berrie, L., Fox, M. P., Gadd, S. C., Harrison, W. J., Keeble, C., Ranker, L. R., Textor, J., Tomova, G. D., Gilthorpe, M. S., & Ellison, G. T. H. (2021). Use of directed acyclic graphs (DAGs) to identify confounders in applied health research: Review and recommendations. *International Journal of Epidemiology*, *50*(2), 620–632. [CrossRef] [PubMed]

Valencia-Ortiz, R., & Cabero-Almenara, J. (2019). La adicción a las redes sociales: Validación de un instrumento en el contexto mexicano [Addiction to social networks: Validation of an instrument in the Mexican context]. *Health and Addictions/Salud y Drogas*, *19*(2), 149–159. [CrossRef]

Vázquez, I. G., Carmona, G. E., Celedonio, F. G. M., Murcia, K. C., Uscanga, R. N. C., & Chagala, A. A. (2025). Asociación de adicción a redes sociales con desempeño académico de estudiantes de enfermería [Association between social media addiction and academic performance among nursing students]. *Ciencia Latina Revista Científica Multidisciplinar*, *9*(2), 4412–4425. [CrossRef]

Vázquez-Salas, A., Hubert, C., Portillo-Romero, A., Valdez-Santiago, R., Barrientos-Gutiérrez, T., & Villalobos, A. (2023). Sintomatología depresiva en adolescentes y adultos mexicanos: Ensanut 2022 [Depressive symptoms among Mexican adolescents and adults: Ensanut 2022]. *Salud Pública de México*, *65*, s117–s125. [CrossRef]

Vo, T. N., Chiu, H.-Y., Chuang, Y.-H., & Huang, H.-C. (2023). Prevalence of stress and anxiety among nursing students: A systematic review and meta-analysis. *Nurse Educator*, *48*(3), E90. [CrossRef]

Wang, J., & Wang, S. (2025). The emotional reinforcement mechanism of and phased intervention strategies for social media addiction. *Behavioral Sciences*, *15*(5), 665. [CrossRef]

Wang, W., Zhu, Y., Yu, H., Wu, C., Li, T., Ji, C., Jiang, Y., & Ding, D. (2024). The impact of sleep quality on emotion regulation difficulties in adolescents: A chained mediation model involving daytime dysfunction, social exclusion, and self-control. *BMC Public Health*, *24*(1), 1862. [CrossRef]

Wang, Y., Guang, Z., Zhang, J., Han, L., Zhang, R., Chen, Y., Chen, Q., Liu, Z., Gao, Y., Wu, R., & Wang, S. (2023). Effect of sleep quality on anxiety and depression symptoms among college students in China's xizang region: The mediating effect of cognitive emotion regulation. *Behavioral Sciences*, *13*(10), 861. [CrossRef] [PubMed]

World Health Organization. (2020, September 18). *State of the world's nursing 2020: Investing in education, jobs and leadership (Annex)* [Web annex]. Available online: https://www.who.int/publications/i/item/9789240007017 (accessed on 11 August 2025).

Yan, N., Long, Y., Yuan, H., Zhou, X., Xie, B., & Wang, Y. (2024). The impact of mobile social media use on depressive mood among college students: A chain mediating effect of upward social comparison and cognitive overload. *Psychology Research and Behavior Management*, *17*, 2111–2120. [CrossRef]

Ye, X., & Gao, H. (2025). Distress disclosure on social media and depressive symptoms among college students: The roles of social comparison and gender. *Frontiers in Psychology*, *16*, 1520066. [CrossRef] [PubMed]

Yu, D. J., Wing, Y. K., Li, T. M. H., & Chan, N. Y. (2024). The impact of social media use on sleep and mental health in youth: A scoping review. *Current Psychiatry Reports*, *26*(3), 104–119. [CrossRef]

Zhang, Y., Jia, X., Yang, Y., Sun, N., Shi, S., & Wang, W. (2024). Change in the global burden of depression from 1990-2019 and its prediction for 2030. *Journal of Psychiatric Research*, *178*, 16–22. [CrossRef] [PubMed]

Zhu, X., Zheng, T., Ding, L., Zhang, X., Li, Z., & Jiang, H. (2023). Exploring associations between social media addiction, social media fatigue, fear of missing out and sleep quality among university students: A cross-section study. *PLoS ONE*, *18*(10), e0292429. [CrossRef] [PubMed]

European Journal of
Investigation in Health, Psychology and Education

MDPI

Article

Association Between Problematic TikTok Use and Procrastination, Loneliness, and Self-Esteem: A Moderation Analysis by Sex and Generation

Aglaia Katsiroumpa [1,*], Zoe Katsiroumpa [1], Evmorfia Koukia [2], Polyxeni Mangoulia [2], Parisis Gallos [3], Ioannis Moisoglou [4] and Petros Galanis [1]

1 Clinical Epidemiology Laboratory, Faculty of Nursing, National and Kapodistrian University of Athens, 11527 Athens, Greece; zkatsiroumpa@nurs.uoa.gr (Z.K.); pegalan@nurs.uoa.gr (P.G.)
2 Laboratory Nursing Counselling and Psychoeducation of Patients and Caregivers, Faculty of Nursing, National and Kapodistrian University of Athens, 11527 Athens, Greece; ekoukia@nurs.uoa.gr (E.K.); pmango@nurs.uoa.gr (P.M.)
3 Faculty of Nursing, University of West Attica, 12243 Athens, Greece; parisgallos@nurs.uoa.gr
4 Faculty of Nursing, University of Thessaly, 41500 Larissa, Greece; iomoysoglou@uth.gr
* Correspondence: aglaiakat@nurs.uoa.gr

Abstract: The aim of this study was to examine the association between problematic TikTok use and procrastination, loneliness, and self-esteem in Greece. Moreover, we performed a moderation analysis to examine potential moderators such as sex and age. We conducted a cross-sectional study with a convenience sample of 1033 TikTok users. We used the TikTok Addiction Scale to measure problematic TikTok use. Additionally, we measured procrastination, loneliness, and self-esteem with the Irrational Procrastination Scale, the UCLA 3-Item Loneliness Scale, and the Rosenberg Self-Esteem Scale, respectively. We performed moderation analysis using linear regression models. We found a positive association between problematic TikTok use, procrastination, and loneliness. Also, we found a negative association between problematic TikTok use and self-esteem. Moderation analysis showed a more prominent association between problematic TikTok use and procrastination among females and Generation Z. The association between problematic TikTok use and loneliness was stronger among males and Generation X. The association between problematic TikTok use and self-esteem was stronger among males and Generation Z. In conclusion, our study supports the negative effect of problematic TikTok use on users. Moreover, sex and gender are moderators in these associations. However, due to study limitations, further research should be conducted.

Keywords: TikTok; procrastination; loneliness; self-esteem; TikTok Addiction Scale; sex; age

1. Introduction

A widely known trait of our times refers to the domination of social media, which spread to high numbers, becoming part of daily life for most of the world, especially for young people (Statista, 2025). Using extremely updated and smart algorithms, social media can easily and in detail "read" their users, figure out their personality, and introduce to them contents of high relevancy to their taste and interest (Kim, 2017; Swart, 2021). According to the statistics, there were 5.44 billion users in 2025, which are expected to rise to 6.46 by the end of 2029 (Statista, 2025).

Among all social media platforms, TikTok is the most prominent one. With the new generations spending most of their day watching videos on TikTok, it is characterized as the most powerful social media platform (Katsiroumpa et al., 2025c; Statista, 2025). TikTok gathers 1.5 billion users monthly, with 35% of its users referring to Generation Z (age group of 16 to 24 years old) (Katsiroumpa et al., 2025c; Statista, 2025). Both statistics and the literature claim that TikTok entails a great load of addiction (Koetsier, 2024; Montag et al., 2021; Pedrouzo & Krynski, 2023). According to United States statistics, there were almost common rates among generations regarding addiction and negative mental health association. More specifically, Generation Z comes first, with 77.7% of them supporting that TikTok seems to be addictive, followed by the Millennials (73.5%) and Gen X (71.7%) (Statista, 2023).

Although the up to 60 s videos that TikTok produce are usually used for casual, harmless reasons (such as informing, promotion, and updates concerning trends) and they can be a potential creative environment for self-expression, the literature claims several concerning issues. First, it is estimated that the time users devote to TikTok may span from 52 to 150 min or more (Statista, 2025; Oberlo, 2023). This fact, along with the psychological effect TikTok reflects on users, raises addiction-related concerns. TikTok follows the exact same pathway as any other addictive habit: the dopaminergic system (Andreassen et al., 2016; Campanella, 2024; Chung, 2018). In fact, TikTok has a double way to allure and conquer its users, first, by providing joy and pleasure to the TikTokers via recognition and, secondly, with the euphoria it brings by the constant consumption of videos highly relevant to users' interests and tastes. One way or another, TikTok engages its users, since both ways lead to the stimulation of the dopaminergic system and the reward mechanism, which is responsible for obtaining pleasure (Koetsier, 2024; Montag et al., 2021). As the individuals try to re-experience the initial pleasure by repeating it, they end up addicted, craving for more (Caponnetto et al., 2025; Koetsier, 2024; Montag et al., 2021). It was indicated that, as per 2023 statistics in a United States survey, participants attributed addictive behaviors towards TikTok and effects on mental health. More specifically, 73.5% of the participants agreed that TikTok is addictive, while 26.8% blamed the platform for negative mental health as a result of TikTok usage (Statista, 2023).

The impact of TikTok on individuals' self-esteem is also very questionable. The term of self-esteem refers to the degree of positive perception of one's image. According to the American Psychological Association "self-esteem reflects a person's physical self-image, view of their accomplishments and capabilities, and values and perceived success in living up to them, as well as the ways in which others view and respond to that person" (American Psychological Association, 2023). Two meta-analyses showed that self-esteem increases as individuals get older. In addition, men tend to have stronger self-esteem than women (Bleidorn et al., 2016; Kling et al., 1999). Concerning TikTok and its relationship to self-esteem, the literature indicates that the impact of unrealistic models and lifestyles that TikTok promotes ends up with self-esteem-related problems for users (Bissonette Mink & Szymanski, 2022; Conte et al., 2025; Galanis et al., 2024a). Studies suggest that women seem to be more burdened with self-esteem issues because of the constant display of ideal, non-realistic standards concerning their image. Even TikTok campaigns regarding the enhancement of self-esteem fail their purpose, ending in worse results concerning self-perception and self-esteem (Bissonette Mink & Szymanski, 2022; Harriger et al., 2023; Ibn Auf et al., 2023; Seekis & Kennedy, 2023).

Another important question is how TikTok isolates its users. It derives from several studies that individuals, and most frequently boys, are feeling uncomfortable and isolated when they are not online and away from social media (including TikTok). More specifically, they declare lack of communication and a feeling of isolation (Conte et al., 2025; Muñoz-Rodríguez et al., 2023; Savoia et al., 2021; Sipal et al., 2011). This finding can be explained in the context of "fear of missing out" phenomenon, where social media and internet users feel that they are missing important information and social updates when they go offline (Bao & Li, 2025; X. Li & Ye, 2022; Wu et al., 2025). These findings show that real-world connection and interpersonal touch seem to be understudied by the digital companion. In addition to the above, the literature supports that loneliness is increased among TikTok users. Either due to total absence of real-world personal relationships or due to poor quality in interpersonal connection, users tend to feel more lonely (Chao et al., 2023; Harries et al., 2025; Huang, 2017; Smith & Short, 2022). Although, studies from the general population show that, as people, especially women, get older, they experience more loneliness (Nicolaisen & Thorsen, 2024; Pagan, 2020; Wang et al., 2023), according to Pop et al., things are reversed, meaning that the younger the users of social media are, the more lonely they feel (Pop et al., 2022).

Studies have supported that social media and mobile phone addiction along with the "fear of missing out" phenomenon have been linked to procrastination especially among young people (Bao & Li, 2025; X. Li & Ye, 2022; Wu et al., 2025). This means that individuals are pushing their responsibilities back in order to spend more time on social media platforms, thinking that, if they do so, they will stay connected to other users and updated (Fuentes Chavez et al., 2025; X. Li & Ye, 2022; Naushad et al., 2025; Zhou et al., 2024). Doomscrolling—the compulsive consumption of negative news on digital platforms—has emerged as a significant contributor to procrastination. Research indicates that individuals often turn to doomscrolling as an avoidance strategy when faced with tasks that evoke stress, boredom, or fear of failure. This behavior provides immediate gratification through novelty and emotional engagement, while the tasks being avoided typically offer delayed rewards. Consequently, doomscrolling not only consumes valuable time but also heightens anxiety and cognitive overload, further impairing focus and productivity. Studies have shown a strong correlation between doomscrolling and procrastination, suggesting that this habit perpetuates a self-reinforcing cycle of avoidance and diminished well-being (Punzalan et al., 2024; Satici et al., 2023; I. M. Hughes et al., 2024). We should mention that TikTok and YouTube Shorts serve similar purposes—short-form video sharing—but their core functions differ significantly. TikTok operates as a standalone platform built entirely around short, trend-driven videos, prioritizing entertainment and rapid content discovery through its highly personalized "For You Page". Its design encourages viral growth and interactive engagement. In contrast, YouTube Shorts is integrated into the broader YouTube ecosystem, functioning as an entry point to long-form content and channel growth. While TikTok focuses on quick, ephemeral trends, YouTube Shorts emphasizes sustained creator development, leveraging searchability, watch time, and monetization. Essentially, TikTok functions as a viral content engine, whereas YouTube Shorts acts as a strategic tool for long-term audience building and monetization. Smartphones and social media have been indicated as responsible not only for "bed-time" but also academic procrastination among students, especially among male students (Naushad et al., 2025). According to studies, self-control seems to play a key role to the limitation of procrastination (Geng et al., 2021; Rasouli et al., 2025). Lastly, smartphone addiction has been correlated to poor mental health such as depression and anxiety due to bed-time procrastination (Geng et al., 2021). Procrastination is a major factor since it is responsible for poor academic and school performance, especially among boys who tend to skip their homework more often than girls (Chao et al., 2023; Rasouli et al., 2025; Sipal et al., 2011; Zacks & Hen, 2018). Furthermore, procrastination has been associated with poor sleep and bad quality of night-time sleep (Hill et al., 2022; Ma et al., 2022).

In brief, research has shown that social media and mobile phone addiction, combined with the fear of missing out, are strongly associated with procrastination, particularly among young people (Bao & Li, 2025; X. Li & Ye, 2022; Wu et al., 2025). However, no studies until now have investigated the association between problematic TikTok use and procrastination. Additionally, the literature regarding the association between problematic TikTok use and self-esteem is limited since only three studies have identified a negative association between these variables (Bissonette Mink & Szymanski, 2022; Conte et al., 2025; Galanis et al., 2024a). In particular, the promotion of unrealistic models and lifestyles on TikTok often leads to self-esteem issues among its users, especially among females. Moreover, limited research indicates that TikTok users experience higher levels of loneliness, often due to a complete lack of real-world personal relationships or the poor quality of their interpersonal connections (Chao et al., 2023; Harries et al., 2025; Huang, 2017; Smith & Short, 2022). In this context, we investigated the association between problematic TikTok use and procrastination, loneliness, and self-esteem. Moreover, we examined the role of sex and age as potential modifiers. In detail, the research hypotheses of this study were the following:

H1. *Problematic TikTok use would be positively associated with procrastination.*

H2. *Sex would moderate the association between problematic TikTok use and procrastination.*

H3. *Age would moderate the association between problematic TikTok use and procrastination.*

H4. *Problematic TikTok use would be positively associated with loneliness.*

H5. *Sex would moderate the association between problematic TikTok use and loneliness.*

H6. *Age would moderate the association between problematic TikTok use and loneliness.*

H7. *Problematic TikTok use would be negatively associated with self-esteem.*

H8. *Sex would moderate the association between problematic TikTok use and self-esteem.*

H9. *Age would moderate the association between problematic TikTok use and self-esteem.*

2. Materials and Methods

2.1. Study Design

We conducted a web-based cross-sectional study in Greece, utilizing an online version of the study questionnaire developed through Google Forms, which was disseminated via TikTok. Data collection occurred from January to March 2025. Specifically, we produced a TikTok video to inform users about our study. Participants were required to be adults over the age of 18. The Google Forms link was sent to interested TikTok users through inbox messages. Prior to commencing the online survey, participants were presented with an introductory page containing essential information. This page detailed the study's purpose and design, provided a brief overview of the questions, estimated the time required to complete the questionnaire, emphasized the voluntary nature of participation, and informed participants of their ability to exit the survey by closing their web browser. Additionally, our contact information was provided to the participants. To ensure data integrity, we inquired whether participants had previously completed the survey, and any affirmative responses were subsequently excluded from the dataset, resulting in a convenience sample. We applied the Reporting of Observational Studies in Epidemiology (STROBE) (Vandenbroucke et al., 2007) to perform our study.

We used G*Power v.3.1.9.2 (Düsseldorf, Germany) to calculate our sample size. Considering a small effect size between problematic TikTok use and procrastination, loneliness, and self-esteem (Cohen's $f^2 = 0.02$), the number of independent variables (one predictor and seven confounders), a confidence level of 99%, and a margin error of 5%, sample size was estimated at 921 participants. Given that the final sample in this study comprised 1033 participants and the calculated effect sizes, the post hoc power was estimated at 99.5%.

2.2. Measurements

We assessed problematic TikTok use using the TikTok Addiction Scale (TTAS), which consists of 15 items and evaluates six dimensions: salience (two items), mood modification (two items), tolerance (three items), withdrawal symptoms (two items), conflict (four items), and relapse (two items) (Galanis et al., 2024c). Salience pertains to users' preoccupation with TikTok, while mood modification refers to its ability to improve emotional well-being. Tolerance is evident when users need to engage more with TikTok to feel satisfied, and withdrawal is characterized by negative feelings when they stop using it. Conflict occurs when TikTok disrupts daily life, while relapse is when users revert to previous usage patterns after abstaining. The TTAS evaluates individuals' attitudes towards TikTok over the past year, with responses on a five-point Likert scale from 1 (very rarely) to 5 (very often). Scores for the TTAS and the six factors range from 1 to 5, with higher scores indicating more problematic TikTok use. The response range for the six subscales ranges from 1 to 5. Also, the response range for the entire scale ranges from 1 to 5. Total score for the entire scale and the subscales is calculated as a mean score of all answers on items. A cut-off score of 3.23 is suggested to differentiate between healthy and problematic users (Galanis et al., 2024b). This cut-off score refers to the mean score of the total scale. The variable that we analyzed is degree of addiction to TikTok (response range from 1 to 5). We used the valid Greek version of the TTAS (Katsiroumpa et al., 2025c). In our study, the TTAS had a Cronbach's alpha of 0.944, and the six factors had Cronbach's alphas ranging from 0.689 to 0.911. Comparative fit index (CFI), Tucker–Lewis index (TLI), and root mean square error of approximation (RMSEA) for the TTAS were 0.984, 0.982, and 0.043, respectively.

We measured procrastination with the Irrational Procrastination Scale (IPS) (Steel, 2010). The IPS includes nine items, such as "I delay tasks beyond what is reasonable" and "I do everything when I believe it needs to be done". Answers are on a five-point Likert scale from 1 (very seldom or not true of me) to 5 (very often true, or true of me). Total score on the IPS ranges from 9 to 45, with higher scores indicating higher levels of procrastination. The variable that we analyzed is degree of procrastination (response range from 9 to 45). We used the valid Greek version of the IPS (Katsiroumpa et al., 2025a). In our study, the TTAS had a Cronbach's alpha of 0.893. CFI, TLI, and RMSEA for the IPS were 0.958, 0.944, and 0.077, respectively.

We measured loneliness with the UCLA 3-Item Loneliness Scale (UCLA-LS-3) (M. E. Hughes et al., 2004). The UCLA-LS-3 includes three items, such as "How often do you feel that you lack companionship?" and "How often do you feel left out?" Answers are on a three-point Likert scale from 1 (hardly ever) to 3 (often). Total score on the UCLA-LS-3 ranges from 3 to 9, with higher scores indicating higher levels of loneliness. The variable that we analyzed is degree of loneliness (response range from 3 to 9). We used the valid Greek version of the UCLA-LS-3 (Katsiroumpa et al., 2025b). In our study, the UCLA-LS-3 had a Cronbach's alpha of 0.807. CFI, TLI, and RMSEA for the UCLA-LS-3 were 0.988, 0.993, and 0.001, respectively.

We measured self-esteem with the Rosenberg Self-Esteem Scale (RSES) (Rosenberg, 1965). The RSES includes 10 items, such as "On the whole, I am satisfied with myself" and "I feel that I have a number of good qualities". Answers are on a four-point Likert scale from 1 (strongly disagree) to 4 (strongly agree). Total score on the RSES ranges from 10 to 40, with higher scores indicating higher levels of self-esteem. The variable that we analyzed is level of self-esteem (response range from 10 to 40). We used the valid Greek version of the RSES (Galanou et al., 2014). In our study, the RSES had a Cronbach's alpha of 0.888. CFI, TLI, and RMSEA for the RSES were 0.995, 0.982, and 0.071, respectively.

We measured the following demographic variables: sex (females or males), age (continuous variable), educational level (elementary school, high school, university degree, MSc diploma, or PhD diploma), socioeconomic status, TikTok use per day (continuous variable), social media use per day (continuous variable), and total number of social media accounts (continuous variable). We categorized our participants into three age generations. In particular, Generation Z referred to people born between 1997 and 2012, Millennials referred to people born between 1981 and 1996, and Generation X referred to people born between 1965 and 1980 (Dimock, 2019). We measured socioeconomic status with a simple question: "How do you consider your socioeconomic status?" Answers were on a scale from 0 to 10, where 0 referred to the worst socioeconomic status and 10 to the best socioeconomic status.

2.3. Participants

Our study population included 1033 participants. Table 1 shows demographic characteristics of our participants. In our sample, 75.4% were females, while 24.6 were males. Mean age was 31.1 years (SD; 12.4), with a median of 26.0 years. Most participants belonged to Generation Z (53.6%), while 28.6% belonged to Millennials and 17.8% belonged to Generation X. Among our participants, 60.4% possessed a university degree, while 39.6% attended high school. The mean value on the socioeconomic status scale denoted a moderate level.

Table 1. Demographic characteristics of our participants (N = 1033).

Characteristics	N	%	95% Confidence Interval
Sex			
Females	779	75.4	72.7 to 78.0
Males	254	24.6	21.9 to 27.3
Age [a]	31.1	12.4	30.4 to 31.9
Age categories			
Generation Z	554	53.6	50.5 to 56.7
Millennials	295	28.6	25.8 to 31.4
Generation X	184	17.8	15.5 to 20.3
Educational level			
High school	409	39.6	36.6 to 42.7
University degree	373	36.1	33.2 to 39.1
MSc diploma	229	22.2	19.7 to 24.8
PhD diploma	22	2.1	1.3 to 3.2
Socioeconomic status [a]	6.2	1.5	6.1 to 6.3

[a] mean, standard deviation.

2.4. Ethical Issues

We conducted our study according to the guidelines of the Declaration of Helsinki (World Medical Association, 2013). Our study protocol was approved by the Ethics Committee of the Faculty of Nursing, National and Kapodistrian University of Athens (approval number; 05, 10 October 2024). Participants were informed about the study design and asked to consent to participate. Specifically, before accessing the online questionnaire, TikTok users were asked via Google Forms if they agreed to participate. Those who consented were allowed to complete the questionnaire, thereby obtaining informed consent. Furthermore, no identifying data were collected from participants, ensuring that participation was both voluntary and anonymous.

2.5. Statistical Analysis

We present categorical variables as numbers (n) and percentages (%) and continuous variables with mean, standard deviation (SD), median, and interquartile range. We used the Kolmogorov–Smirnov test and Q-Q plots to assess the distribution of continuous variables. We considered TikTok addiction as the independent variable. We found moderate to high correlations between the six factors on the TTAS since correlation coefficients ranged from 0.554 to 0.771 (p-value < 0.001 in all cases). Thus, to avoid multicollinearity in the multivariable regression models, we chose to use the total score on the TTAS as the independent variable. Our dependent variables were procrastination, loneliness, and self-esteem scores. Demographic and social media characteristics were considered as potential confounders. We performed moderation analysis (Hair et al., 2021) to examine if sex and age are moderators in the association between problematic TikTok use and procrastination, loneliness, and self-esteem. We centered the independent variable (TTAS score) and the moderator variable (age) to reduce multicollinearity (Iacobucci et al., 2017). For instance, "centered" variable of TTAS score was obtained by subtracting the mean TTAS score from each individual TTAS score value. Similarly, we calculated the "centered" variable of age. Since the dependent variables were continuous and normally distributed, we applied linear regression analysis, presenting unstandardized and standardized coefficients beta, 95% confidence intervals (CI), and p-values. First, we created a linear regression model including the independent variable (TTAS score) and the moderator (sex or age). Then, we created a second regression by adding the interaction term (TTAS score ∗ sex or age). We calculated the total variance (R^2) of the dependent variable explained in the two models. Statistically significant coefficients beta for the interaction term indicated the presence of moderation. Moreover, we performed simple slope analysis to identify the direction of the moderating effects introduced by sex and age. p-values less than 0.05 were considered statistically significant. We used the IBM SPSS 28.0 (IBM Corp. Released 2021. IBM SPSS Statistics for Windows, Version 28.0. Armonk, NY, USA, IBM Corp.) for analysis.

3. Results

3.1. Social Media Characteristics

Mean TikTok use per day was 1.8 h (SD, 1.5), with a median of 1 hour, a minimum value of 30 min, and a maximum value of 8.0 h. Mean TikTok use per day was 1.8 h (SD, 1.5) for females and 1.7 h (SD, 1.5) for males. Mean TikTok use per day was 2.3 h (SD, 1.7) for Generation Z, 1.3 h (SD, 1.1) for Millennials, and 0.8 h (SD, 0.5) for Generation X.

The mean social media use per day was 3.3 h (SD, 1.9), with a median of 3.0 h, a minimum value of 30 min, and a maximum value of 8.0 h. Mean social media use per day was 3.4 h (SD, 1.9) for females and 3.3 h (SD, 1.8) for males. Mean social media use per day was 4.0 h (SD, 1.8) for Generation Z, 2.9 h (SD, 1.7) for Millennials, and 2.1 h (SD, 1.4) for Generation X.

Most participants (92.9%, n = 960) had accounts on at least two social media platforms. In particular, 7.1% (n = 73) had an account only on TikTok, 15.8% (n = 163) had accounts on two social media platforms, 28.0% (n = 289) on three social media platforms, 21.9% (n = 226) on four social media platforms, 15.4% (n = 159) on five social media platforms, and 11.9%

(n = 123) on 6–8 social media platforms. Mean number of accounts was 3.6 (SD; 1.5), with a median of 3.0, a minimum value of 1, and a maximum value of 8.

3.2. Association Between Problematic TikTok Use and Procrastination with Sex as the Moderator

Table 2 presents moderation analysis with procrastination score as the dependent variable and sex as the moderator. The first regression model, which included the independent variable (centered TikTok addiction score) and the moderator (sex), explained 32.1% of the variance in procrastination score (R^2 = 32.1%, *p*-value < 0.001). The second regression model, which added the interaction term (TikTok addiction score ∗ sex), explained an additional 0.4% of the variance (ΔR^2 = 0.4%, *p*-value = 0.013), bringing the total variance explained to 32.5% (R^2 = 32.5%, *p*-value < 0.001). In the first model, TikTok addiction score had a significant effect on procrastination. We found a positive association between TikTok addiction score and procrastination. In the second model, both TikTok addiction score and sex remained significant, and the interaction term also significantly predicted procrastination. Thus, sex moderated the association between TikTok addiction score and procrastination. Simple slopes analysis indicated a stronger association between TikTok addiction score and procrastination among females (Figure 1).

Table 2. Moderation analysis (linear regression models) with procrastination score as the dependent variable and sex as the moderator.

	Unstandardized Coefficient Beta	95% CI for Beta	Standardized Coefficient Beta	*p*-Value	Adjusted R^2 (%)
Model 1					32.1
TikTok addiction score	5.206	4.743 to 5.660	0.566	<0.001	
Sex	0.739	0.119 to 1.597	0.043	0.014	
Model 2					32.5
TikTok addiction score	5.560	5.019 to 6.100	0.604	<0.001	
Sex	3.331	1.108 to 5.553	0.195	0.003	
Interaction TikTok addiction score ∗ sex	−1.317	−2.360 to −0.275	−0.170	0.013	

CI: confidence interval.

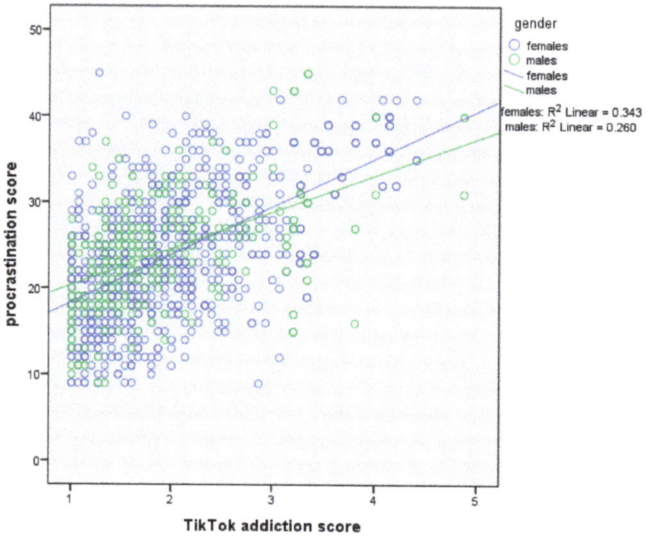

Figure 1. Simple slopes analysis with procrastination score as the dependent variable and sex as the moderator.

3.3. Association Between Problematic TikTok Use and Procrastination with Age as the Moderator

Table 3 presents moderation analysis with procrastination score as the dependent variable and age as the moderator. The first regression model, which included the independent variable (centered TikTok addiction score) and the moderator (age), explained 36.2% of the variance in procrastination score (R^2 = 36.2%, *p*-value < 0.001). The second regression model, which added the interaction term (TikTok addiction score ∗ age), explained an additional 0.6% of the variance (ΔR^2 = 0.4%, *p*-value = 0.011), bringing the total variance explained to 36.8% (R^2 = 36.8%, *p*-value < 0.001). In the first model, TikTok addiction score had a significant effect on procrastination. We found a positive association between TikTok addiction score and procrastination. In the second model, both TikTok addiction score and age remained significant, and the interaction term also significantly predicted procrastination. Thus, age moderated the association between TikTok addiction score and procrastination. Simple slopes analysis indicated a stronger association between TikTok addiction score and procrastination in Generation Z (Figure 2).

Table 3. Moderation analysis (linear regression models) with procrastination score as the dependent variable and age as the moderator.

	Unstandardized Coefficient Beta	95% CI for Beta	Standardized Coefficient Beta	*p*-Value	Adjusted R^2 (%)
Model 1					36.2
TikTok addiction score	5.596	5.069 to 6.124	0.591	<0.001	
Age	−0.183	−0.219 to −0.148	−0.300	<0.001	
Model 2					36.8
TikTok addiction score	5.208	4.583 to 5.834	0.550	<0.001	
Age	−0.039	−0.078 to −0.012	−0.063	0.041	
Interaction TikTok addiction score ∗ age	−0.061	−0.114 to −0.008	−0.069	0.024	

CI: confidence interval.

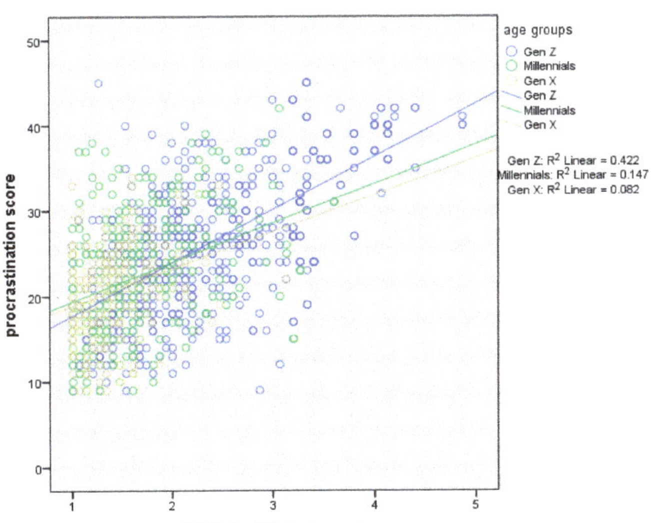

Figure 2. Simple slopes analysis with procrastination score as the dependent variable and age as the moderator.

3.4. Association Between Problematic TikTok Use and Loneliness with Sex as the Moderator

Table 4 presents moderation analysis with loneliness score as the dependent variable and sex as the moderator. The first regression model, which included the independent variable (centered TikTok addiction score) and the moderator (sex), explained 16.9% of the variance in loneliness score (R^2 = 16.9%, *p*-value < 0.001). The second regression model, which added the interaction term (TikTok addiction score ∗ sex), explained an additional 0.4% of the variance (ΔR^2 = 0.4%, *p*-value = 0.015), bringing the total variance explained to 17.3% (R^2 = 17.3%, *p*-value < 0.001). In the first model, TikTok addiction score had a significant effect on loneliness. We found a positive association between TikTok addiction score and loneliness. In the second model, both TikTok addiction score and sex remained significant, and the interaction term also significantly predicted loneliness. Thus, sex moderated the association between TikTok addiction score and loneliness. Simple slopes analysis indicated a stronger association between TikTok addiction score and loneliness among males (Figure 3).

Table 4. Moderation analysis (linear regression models) with loneliness score as the dependent variable and sex as the moderator.

	Unstandardized Coefficient Beta	95% CI for Beta	Standardized Coefficient Beta	*p*-Value	Adjusted R^2 (%)
Model 1					16.9
TikTok addiction score	0.940	0.813 to 1.066	0.413	<0.001	
Sex	−0.888	−1.256 to −0.243	−0.213	0.008	
Model 2					17.3
TikTok addiction score	0.845	0.697 to 0.992	0.371	<0.001	
Sex	−0.807	−1.415 to −0.199	−0.191	0.009	
Interaction TikTok addiction score ∗ sex	0.353	0.068 to 0.638	0.184	0.015	

CI: confidence interval.

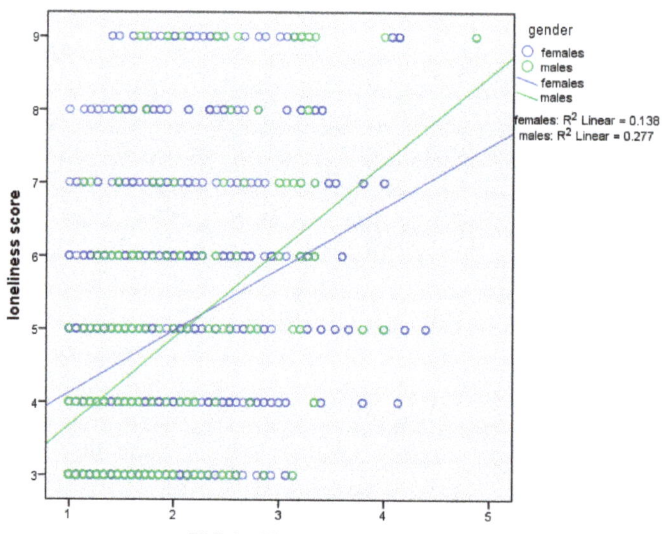

Figure 3. Simple slopes analysis with loneliness score as the dependent variable and sex as the moderator.

3.5. Association Between Problematic TikTok Use and Loneliness with Age as the Moderator

Table 5 presents moderation analysis with loneliness score as the dependent variable and age as the moderator. The first regression model, which included the independent variable (centered TikTok addiction score) and the moderator (age), explained 16.9% of the variance in loneliness score (R^2 = 16.9%, p-value < 0.001). The second regression model, which added the interaction term (TikTok addiction score ∗ age), explained an additional 1.3% of the variance (ΔR^2 = 1.3%, p-value < 0.001), bringing the total variance explained to 18.2% (R^2 = 18.2%, p-value < 0.001). In the first model, TikTok addiction score had a significant effect on loneliness. We found a positive association between TikTok addiction score and loneliness. In the second model, both TikTok addiction score and age remained significant, and the interaction term also significantly predicted loneliness. Thus, age moderated the association between TikTok addiction score and loneliness. Simple slopes analysis indicated a stronger association between TikTok addiction score and procrastination in Generation X (Figure 4).

Table 5. Moderation analysis (linear regression models) with loneliness score as the dependent variable and age as the moderator.

	Unstandardized Coefficient Beta	95% CI for Beta	Standardized Coefficient Beta	p-Value	Adjusted R^2 (%)
Model 1					16.9
TikTok addiction score	0.921	0.776 to 1.065	0.405	<0.001	
Age	0.034	0.022 to 0.042	0.211	<0.001	
Model 2					18.2
TikTok addiction score	1.116	0.946 to 1.286	0.490	<0.001	
Age	0.024	0.012 to 0.046	0.189	<0.001	
Interaction TikTok addiction score ∗ age	0.031	0.016 to 0.045	0.145	<0.001	

CI: confidence interval.

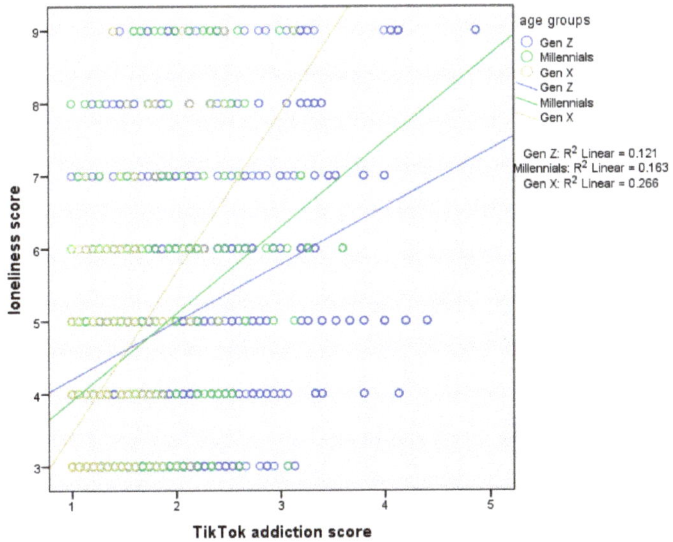

Figure 4. Simple slopes analysis with loneliness score as the dependent variable and age as the moderator.

3.6. Association Between Problematic TikTok Use and Self-Esteem with Sex as the Moderator

Table 6 presents moderation analysis with self-esteem score as the dependent variable and sex as the moderator. The first regression model, which included the independent variable (centered TikTok addiction score) and the moderator (sex), explained 16.4% of the variance in self-esteem score (R^2 = 16.4%, *p*-value < 0.001). The second regression model, which added the interaction term (TikTok addiction score ∗ sex), explained an additional 0.7% of the variance (ΔR^2 = 0.7%, *p*-value = 0.003), bringing the total variance explained to 17.1% (R^2 = 17.1%, *p*-value < 0.001). In the first model, TikTok addiction score had a significant effect on self-esteem. We found a negative association between TikTok addiction score and self-esteem. In the second model, both TikTok addiction score and sex remained significant, and the interaction term also significantly predicted self-esteem. Thus, sex moderated the association between TikTok addiction score and self-esteem. Simple slopes analysis indicated a stronger association between TikTok addiction score and self-esteem among males (Figure 5).

Table 6. Moderation analysis (linear regression models) with self-esteem score as the dependent variable and sex as the moderator.

	Unstandardized Coefficient Beta	95% CI for Beta	Standardized Coefficient Beta	*p*-Value	Adjusted R^2 (%)
Model 1					16.4
TikTok addiction score	−2.784	−3.168 to −2.400	−0.406	<0.001	
Sex	2.878	0.913 to 4.792	0.236	<0.001	
Model 2					17.1
TikTok addiction score	−2.436	−2.883 to −1.989	−0.355	<0.001	
Sex	2.724	0.885 to 4.563	0.214	0.004	
Interaction TikTok addiction score ∗ sex	−1.298	−2.160 to −0.435	0.003	0.015	

CI: confidence interval.

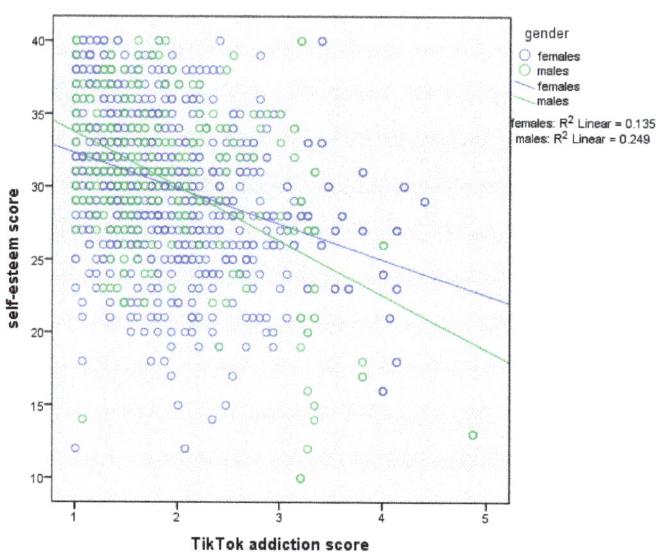

Figure 5. Simple slopes analysis with self-esteem score as the dependent variable and sex as the moderator.

3.7. Association Between Problematic TikTok Use and Self-Esteem with Age as the Moderator

Table 7 presents moderation analysis with self-esteem score as the dependent variable and age as the moderator. The first regression model, which included the independent variable (centered TikTok addiction score) and the moderator (age), explained 18.4% of the variance in self-esteem score (R^2 = 18.4%, *p*-value < 0.001). The second regression model, which added the interaction term (TikTok addiction score ∗ age), explained an additional 0.4% of the variance (ΔR^2 = 0.4%, *p*-value = 0.024), bringing the total variance explained to 18.8% (R^2 = 18.8%, *p*-value < 0.001). In the first model, TikTok addiction score had a significant effect on self-esteem. We found a negative association between TikTok addiction score and self-esteem. In the second model, both TikTok addiction score and age remained significant, and the interaction term also significantly predicted self-esteem. Thus, age moderated the association between TikTok addiction score and self-esteem. Simple slopes analysis indicated a stronger association between TikTok addiction score and self-esteem in Generation Z (Figure 6).

Table 7. Moderation analysis (linear regression models) with self-esteem score as the dependent variable and age as the moderator.

	Unstandardized Coefficient Beta	95% CI for Beta	Standardized Coefficient Beta	*p*-Value	Adjusted R^2 (%)
Model 1					18.4
TikTok addiction score	−2.228	−2.660 to −1.796	−0.325	<0.001	
Age	0.074	0.046 to 0.102	0.168	<0.001	
Model 2					18.8
TikTok addiction score	−1.910	−2.422 to −1.398	−0.278	<0.001	
Age	0.094	0.061 to 0.127	0.213	<0.001	
Interaction TikTok addiction score ∗ age	0.050	0.007 to 0.094	0.079	0.024	

CI: confidence interval.

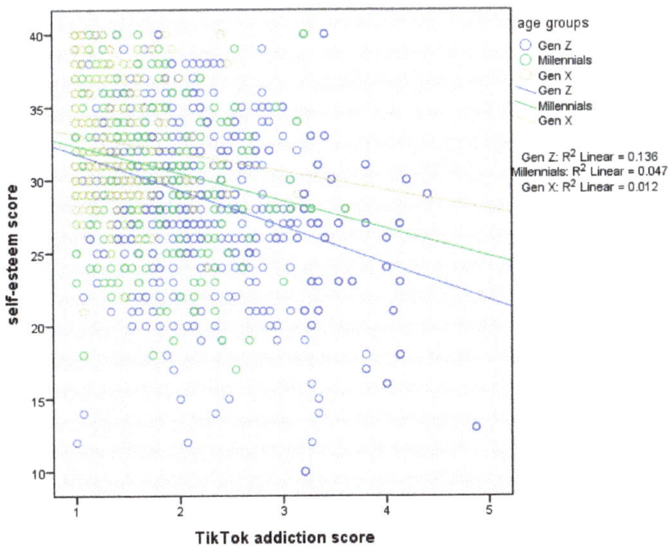

Figure 6. Simple slopes analysis with self-esteem score as the dependent variable and age as the moderator.

4. Discussion

TikTok daily use seems to have steady growth, largely among young generations. This immense spread underlines the major need for further investigation of TikTok's reflection on individuals' health status. Since the literature on this field is scarce, we examined the association between problematic TikTok use, procrastination, loneliness, and self-esteem.

Concerning daily use of TikTok, the sample had a mean time of use of 1.8 h. This finding aligns with other statistical sources concerning time on TikTok, which declare that the time users devote to TikTok may span from 52 to 150 min or more (Oberlo, 2023; Statista, 2025). Female and male participants spent almost the same time on TikTok daily, while, among generations, it was shown that first comes Generation Z, followed by the Millennials and, last, Generation X. These results agree with general statistics, supporting that two genders share almost equal time on TikTok, with Generation Z having the largest period daily (Oberlo, 2023; Statista, 2025). It is of great interest that the mean daily use of social media in this study was 3.3 h; since the mean for TikTok daily use was found to be 1.8 h, it means that the participants devote more than half of their social media time to TikTok. Although 92.9% of the sample had at least two more accounts on other social media, they preferred spending more time on TikTok. This finding verifies previous studies and statistics, which support that TikTok has prevailed over other social media, proving itself more interesting and addictive in contrast to other social media platforms (Wallaroomedia, 2024).

According to our results, there was a positive association between TikTok addiction score and procrastination score especially among females and Generation Z. These results indicate that, the more time is spent on TikTok, the more the users push their real-world responsibilities to the background of priorities. Generation Z is the one with the highest levels of TikTok use daily among all other generations. Furthermore, it is supported that women tend to procrastinate more than men due to a variety of reasons, such as stress, ideal standards of perfection, etc. (Balkis & Duru, 2024; Flett et al., 2016; Niermann & Scheres, 2014). As the literature supports, procrastination occurs either by failing to self-regulate or because of fear of missing out. Either way, users ignore their responsibilities and prioritize their time on TikTok and social media (Bao & Li, 2025; X. Li & Ye, 2022). The literature has underlined that procrastination associated with social media addiction frequently leads to poor sleep (Hale & Guan, 2015) and poor academic and school performance (Chao et al., 2023; Naushad et al., 2025; Zhou et al., 2024; Rasouli et al., 2025).

Another finding was that our sample indicated a positive association between TikTok addiction score and loneliness score. This association was more prominent among males and Generation X. Generation X finds TikTok addictive, ending up "absorbed" (Statista, 2023). Both social media and TikTok, according to other studies, have been associated with negative consequences for users, leading to poor mental health, such as loneliness, depression, stress, and poor sleep (Conte et al., 2025; Muñoz-Rodríguez et al., 2023; Harries et al., 2025; Chao et al., 2023). According to other studies, individuals, and most frequently boys, are feeling isolated when they go offline and especially when they are away from social media (including TikTok), declaring lack of communication and a feeling of isolation (Conte et al., 2025; Muñoz-Rodríguez et al., 2023; Savoia et al., 2021; Sipal et al., 2011). This feeling is attributed to the "fear of missing out" phenomenon, where individuals fear that they are missing important information and social updates when they go offline (Bao & Li, 2025; X. Li & Ye, 2022; Wu et al., 2025). Yet, this absorbance in the digital world costs a great load of real-world communication and interaction.

Moreover, our results indicated a negative association between TikTok addiction and self-esteem. This association was more prominent among males and Generation Z. This finding comes to be added to in the general context that TikTok affects mental health negatively, including self-esteem. More specifically, it is supported that prolonged TikTok use leads users to immerse themselves in a digital world where unrealistic body and lifestyle standards dominate. This daily interaction with non-achievable standards and stereotypes drives them to self-esteem issues, body dissatisfaction, and damaged self-perception (Calogero et al., 2011). Self-esteem issues due to addictive use of TikTok have also derived from Conte et al.'s systematic review where TikTok has been appointed as a risk factor for poor mental health, body-image issues, and low self-esteem (Conte et al., 2025). Both our study and previous studies in the literature support that younger ages are more vulnerable to self-esteem issues, especially when it comes to TikTok (Statista, 2023; Chung, 2018; Bleidorn et al., 2016). Concerning self-esteem and gender, the literature is divided into two parts. Generally, women seem to be more burdened with self-esteem issues due to social and mental-related reasons; yet there are studies supporting that men suffer too from the social stereotypes, leading to low self-esteem (Bleidorn et al., 2016; Casale, 2020; Jouini et al., 2018; Kling et al., 1999; J. Li et al., 2022; Mayo, 2016; Roberts, 1991).

Our study had several limitations. First, we used a convenience sample of TikTok users in Greece. Although we covered the sample size requirements, our sample cannot be representative of TikTok users. Moreover, sampling through TikTok inbox messages may raise self-selection bias. It is probable that participants that share significant characteristics may participate in our study. For instance, our study included mainly females (75.4%) and Generation Z participants (53.6%) and, thus, this sex and age imbalance may introduce selection bias. This selection bias limits generalizability of our findings. Future studies should include random samples to produce more representative results. Second, we conducted a cross-sectional study and, therefore, we cannot establish a causal relationship between problematic TikTok use, procrastination, loneliness, and self-esteem. Thus, we cannot be sure whether problematic TikTok use affects procrastination, loneliness, and self-esteem or whether these variables pre-exist and lead to increased problematic TikTok use. Longitudinal studies that explore the association between problematic TikTok use, procrastination, loneliness, and self-esteem could add significant information. Third, we used valid tools to measure problematic TikTok use, procrastination, loneliness, and self-esteem. However, our participants may compromise their answers due to social desirability bias. Therefore, information bias is probable in our study. Moreover, information bias may be introduced by the measurement of confounders. For instance, we measured socioeconomic status through a self-reported assessment. Fourth, we eliminated several confounders in our study, such as sex, age, educational level, socioeconomic status, TikTok use per day, social media use per day, and social media accounts. However, several other variables may introduce confounding in the association between problematic TikTok use, procrastination, loneliness, and self-esteem. In this context, scholars should eliminate more confounders in future studies. For instance, personality characteristics, family member relationships, and sleep patterns may be considered as potential confounders. Also, mental health issues, psychiatric history, and pre-existing conditions should be considered as potential confounders in future research. Moreover, we used four different length and valid scales to measure problematic TikTok use, procrastination, loneliness, and self-esteem in this study. Therefore, it was difficult to use more scales to measure our confounders since more questions may reduce participation rate. For instance, we measured socioeconomic status via a single self-report item and, thus, information bias is probably introduced in this study. Future studies could use more valid and extended tools to measure confounders such as socioeconomic status. Additionally, investigation of potential mediators in the association between problematic TikTok use, procrastination, loneliness, and self-esteem may further add significant knowledge on the impact of TikTok use. Finally, our scales showed very good Cronbach's alpha, but they are still self-report scales and, thus, information bias is probable. We should mention that Cronbach's alpha for one subscale of the TTAS was 0.689, slightly lower than the value of 0.7. Scholars should obtain in the future more valid measurements of variables such as TikTok use, procrastination, loneliness, and self-esteem to reduce information bias.

5. Conclusions

This study aimed to enlighten and contribute to further understanding of TikTok and its consequences. Interventions should be taken into consideration, in order to reduce the negative effect of problematic TikTok use on mental health. Problematic TikTok use is a modifiable risk factor for poor mental health outcomes. In this context, skills-based micro-interventions, screen-time reduction with sleep safeguards, digital literacy with active mediation, and platform measures may improve intentional use and elevate high-quality content (Herriman et al., 2025). Policy makers, stakeholders, and healthcare professionals can mount an effective, ethical, and scalable response by combining these elements in programs with rigorous monitoring and continuous improvement. Additionally, there is a need for digital/media literacy with active parental/educator mediation for youth and platform features that nudge breaks, elevate evidence-based content, and provide transparent well-being tools (Plackett et al., 2023).

At the individual level, to deal with problematic TikTok use, users can use built-in screen time limits and schedule specific times for app use rather than scrolling impulsively. Also, they can incorporate alternative activities like exercise, hobbies, or socializing offline to replace excessive screen time (Pieh et al., 2025). If TikTok use interferes with sleep, users can enable "do not disturb" mode and avoid the app at least an hour before bedtime. For persistent difficulties, users should consider behavioral strategies such as cognitive restructuring or seek professional support. Finally, users can curate their feed by unfollowing harmful content and engaging with positive, evidence-based creators to make their experience healthier and more intentional (Radtke et al., 2021).

The present study faced a number of limitations, such as the cross-sectional nature of data, and, thus, the findings should be examined under strict scrutiny. Further investigations should be carried out, such as longitudinal studies, to reduce bias and improve knowledge and research in this field.

Author Contributions: Conceptualization, A.K. and P.G. (Petros Galanis); methodology, A.K., I.M. and P.G. (Petros Galanis); software, P.G. (Parisis Gallos) and P.G. (Petros Galanis); validation, Z.K., E.K., P.M. and I.M.; formal analysis, P.G. (Parisis Gallos) and P.G. (Petros Galanis); investigation, A.K., Z.K., E.K., P.M. and I.M.; resources, A.K., Z.K., E.K., P.M. and I.M.; data curation, I.M., P.G. (Parisis Gallos), Z.K., E.K. and P.M.; writing—original draft preparation, A.K., I.M., Z.K., E.K., P.M., P.G. (Parisis Gallos) and P.G. (Petros Galanis); writing—review and editing, A.K., I.M., Z.K., E.K., P.M., P.G. (Parisis Gallos) and P.G. (Petros Galanis); visualization, A.K. and P.G. (Petros Galanis.; supervision, P.G. (Petros Galanis); project administration, A.K. and P.G. (Petros Galanis). All authors have read and agreed to the published version of the manuscript.

Funding: This research received no external funding.

Institutional Review Board Statement: This study was conducted in accordance with the Declaration of Helsinki and approved by the Ethics Committee of the Faculty of Nursing, National and Kapodistrian University of Athens (approval number 05, 10 October 2024).

Informed Consent Statement: Informed consent was obtained from all subjects involved in the study.

Data Availability Statement: The original data presented in this study are openly available in FigShare at doi.org/10.6084/m9.figshare.28903820.

Conflicts of Interest: The authors declare no conflicts of interest.

Abbreviations

The following abbreviations are used in this manuscript:

CFI	Comparative fit index
CI	Confidence interval
IPS	Irrational Procrastination Scale
RMSEA	Root mean square error of approximation
RSES	Rosenberg Self-Esteem Scale
TLI	Tucker–Lewis index
TTAS	TikTok Addiction Scale
UCLA-LS-3	UCLA 3-Item Loneliness Scale

References

American Psychological Association. (2023). *APA dictionary of psychology*. American Psychological Association. Available online: https://dictionary.apa.org/ (accessed on 17 August 2025).

Andreassen, C. S., Billieux, J., Griffiths, M. D., Kuss, D. J., Demetrovics, Z., Mazzoni, E., & Pallesen, S. (2016). The relationship between addictive use of social media and video games and symptoms of psychiatric disorders: A large-scale cross-sectional study. *Psychology of Addictive Behaviors*, *30*(2), 252–262. [CrossRef]

Balkis, M., & Duru, E. (2024). Gender differences in procrastination and subjective well-being: A cross-sectional study among students and non-students. *Psychological Reports, under press*. [CrossRef]

Bao, H., & Li, S. (2025). Self-efficacy, fear of missing out, social media use, and bedtime procrastination in Chinese college students. *Psychological Reports, under press*. [CrossRef]

Bissonette Mink, D., & Szymanski, D. M. (2022). TikTok use and body dissatisfaction: Examining direct, indirect, and moderated relations. *Body Image*, *43*, 205–216. [CrossRef]

Bleidorn, W., Arslan, R. C., Denissen, J. J. A., Rentfrow, P. J., Gebauer, J. E., Potter, J., & Gosling, S. D. (2016). Age and gender differences in self-esteem—A cross-cultural window. *Journal of Personality and Social Psychology*, *111*(3), 396–410. [CrossRef]

Calogero, R. M., Tantleff-Dunn, S., & Thompson, J. K. (2011). *Self-objectification in women: Causes, consequences, and counteractions* (1st ed.). American Psychological Association.

Campanella, S. (2024). Addictive behaviors: Decades of research, but still so many questions! *Frontiers in Psychology*, *15*, 1485118. [CrossRef]

Caponnetto, P., Lanzafame, I., Prezzavento, G. C., Rawashdeh, S., Moussa, M. A., & Fakhrou, A. (2025). Understanding problematic TikTok use: A systematic review of emerging diagnostic and therapeutic implications in clinical psychology. *Journal of Addictive Diseases*, 1–22. [CrossRef] [PubMed]

Casale, S. (2020). Gender differences in self-esteem and self-confidence. In B. J. Carducci, C. S. Nave, A. Fabio, D. H. Saklofske, & C. Stough (Eds.), *The Wiley encyclopedia of personality and individual differences* (pp. 185–189). Wiley. [CrossRef]

Chao, M., Lei, J., He, R., Jiang, Y., & Yang, H. (2023). TikTok use and psychosocial factors among adolescents: Comparisons of non-users, moderate users, and addictive users. *Psychiatry Research*, *325*, 115247. [CrossRef] [PubMed]

Chung, T. (2018). Psychology of addictive behaviors. *Psychology of Addictive Behaviors*, *32*(8), 859–860. [CrossRef]

Conte, G., Iorio, G. D., Esposito, D., Romano, S., Panvino, F., Maggi, S., Altomonte, B., Casini, M. P., Ferrara, M., & Terrinoni, A. (2025). Scrolling through adolescence: A systematic review of the impact of TikTok on adolescent mental health. *European Child & Adolescent Psychiatry*, *34*(5), 1511–1527. [CrossRef]

Dimock, M. (2019). *Defining generations: Where Millennials end and Generation Z begins*. Pew Research Center. Available online: https://www.pewresearch.org/short-reads/2019/01/17/where-millennials-end-and-generation-z-begins/ (accessed on 29 August 2025).

Flett, A. L., Haghbin, M., & Pychyl, T. A. (2016). Procrastination and depression from a cognitive perspective: An exploration of the associations among procrastinatory automatic thoughts, rumination, and mindfulness. *Journal of Rational-Emotive & Cognitive-Behavior Therapy*, *34*(3), 169–186. [CrossRef]

Fuentes Chavez, S. E., Vera-Calmet, V. G., Aguilar-Armas, H. M., Yglesias Alva, L. A., Arbulú Ballesteros, M. A., & Alegria Silva, C. E. (2025). Social media addiction and procrastination in Peruvian university students: Exploring the role of emotional regulation and age moderation. *Healthcare, 13*(9), 1072. [CrossRef]

Galanis, P., Katsiroumpa, A., Katsiroumpa, Z., Mangoulia, P., Gallos, P., Moisoglou, I., & Koukia, E. (2024a). Association between problematic TikTok use and mental health: A systematic review and meta-analysis. *AIMS Public Health, 12*(2), 491–519. [CrossRef] [PubMed]

Galanis, P., Katsiroumpa, A., Moisoglou, I., & Konstantakopoulou, O. (2024b). Determining an optimal cut-off point for TikTok addiction using the TikTok Addiction Scale. *Archives of Hellenic Medicine, 42*(4), 554–559.

Galanis, P., Katsiroumpa, A., Moisoglou, I., & Konstantakopoulou, O. (2024c). The TikTok Addiction Scale: Development and validation. *AIMS Public Health, 11*(4), 1172–1197. [CrossRef]

Galanou, C., Galanakis, M., Alexopoulos, E., & Darviri, C. (2014). Rosenberg Self-Esteem Scale Greek validation on student sample. *Psychology, 5*(8), 819–827. [CrossRef]

Geng, Y., Gu, J., Wang, J., & Zhang, R. (2021). Smartphone addiction and depression, anxiety: The role of bedtime procrastination and self-control. *Journal of Affective Disorders, 293*, 415–421. [CrossRef]

Hair, J. F., Hult, G. T. M., Ringle, C. M., Sarstedt, M., Danks, N. P., & Ray, S. (2021). Moderation analysis. In *Partial least squares structural equation modeling (PLS-SEM) using R*. Classroom companion: Business. Springer. [CrossRef]

Hale, L., & Guan, S. (2015). Screen time and sleep among school-aged children and adolescents: A systematic literature review. *Sleep Medicine Reviews, 21*, 50–58. [CrossRef]

Harries, B., Zenone, M., & Hartwell, G. (2025). Feeling lonely in the online crowd: What TikTok tells us about young people and loneliness. *Health Promotion International, 40*(4), daaf094. [CrossRef]

Harriger, J. A., Wick, M. R., Sherline, C. M., & Kunz, A. L. (2023). The body positivity movement is not all that positive on TikTok: A content analysis of body positive TikTok videos. *Body Image, 46*, 256–264. [CrossRef]

Herriman, Z., Roberts, R. M., Taylor, A. M., & Slater, A. (2025). A cognitive behavioral therapy-based microintervention to reduce the negative impact of Instagram use on well-being: A randomized controlled trial. *Psychology of Popular Media, under press*. [CrossRef]

Hill, V. M., Rebar, A. L., Ferguson, S. A., Shriane, A. E., & Vincent, G. E. (2022). Go to bed! A systematic review and meta-analysis of bedtime procrastination correlates and sleep outcomes. *Sleep Medicine Reviews, 66*, 101697. [CrossRef] [PubMed]

Huang, C. (2017). Time spent on social network sites and psychological well-being: A meta-analysis. *Cyberpsychology, Behavior, and Social Networking, 20*(6), 346–354. [CrossRef] [PubMed]

Hughes, I. M., Keith, M. G., Lee, J., & Gray, C. E. (2024). Working, scrolling, and worrying: Doomscrolling at work and its implications for work engagement. *Computers in Human Behavior, 153*, 108130. [CrossRef]

Hughes, M. E., Waite, L. J., Hawkley, L. C., & Cacioppo, J. T. (2004). A short scale for measuring loneliness in large surveys: Results from two population-based studies. *Research on Aging, 26*(6), 655–672. [CrossRef]

Iacobucci, D., Schneider, M. J., Popovich, D. L., & Bakamitsos, G. A. (2017). Mean centering, multicollinearity, and moderators in multiple regression: The reconciliation redux. *Behavior Research Methods, 49*(1), 403–404. [CrossRef]

Ibn Auf, A. I. A. A., Alblowi, Y. H., Alkhaldi, R. O., Thabet, S. A., Alabdali, A. A. H., Binshalhoub, F. H., Alzahrani, K. A. S., & Alzahrani, R. A. I. (2023). Social comparison and body image in teenage users of the TikTok app. *Cureus, 15*(11), e48227. [CrossRef] [PubMed]

Jouini, E., Karehnke, P., & Napp, C. (2018). Stereotypes, underconfidence and decision-making with an application to gender and math. *Journal of Economic Behavior & Organization, 148*, 34–45. [CrossRef]

Katsiroumpa, A., Katsiroumpa, Z., Koukia, E., Mangoulia, P., Gallos, P., Moisoglou, I., & Galanis, P. (2025a). Irrational Procrastination Scale: Translation and validation in Greek. *International Journal of Caring Sciences, 18*(1), 543–550.

Katsiroumpa, A., Katsiroumpa, Z., Koukia, E., Mangoulia, P., Gallos, P., Moisoglou, I., & Galanis, P. (2025b). UCLA 3-item loneliness scale: Translation and validation in Greek. *International Journal of Caring Sciences, 18*(1), 534–542.

Katsiroumpa, A., Moisoglou, I., Gallos, P., Katsiroumpa, Z., Konstantakopoulou, O., Tsiachri, M., & Galanis, P. (2025c). Problematic TikTok use and its association with poor sleep: A cross-sectional study among Greek young adults. *Psychiatry International, 6*(1), 25. [CrossRef]

Kim, S. A. (2017). Social media algorithms: Why you see what you see technology explainers. *Georgetown Law Technology Review, 2*(1), 147–154.

Kling, K. C., Hyde, J. S., Showers, C. J., & Buswell, B. N. (1999). Gender differences in self-esteem: A meta-analysis. *Psychological Bulletin, 125*(4), 470–500. [CrossRef]

Koetsier, J. (2024). *Digital crack cocaine: The science behind TikTok's success*. Forbes. Available online: https://www.forbes.com/sites/johnkoetsier/2020/01/18/digital-crack-cocaine-the-science-behind-tiktoks-success/ (accessed on 26 August 2025).

Li, J., Liu, Y., & Song, J. (2022). The relationship between gender self-stereotyping and life satisfaction: The mediation role of relational self-esteem and personal self-esteem. *Frontiers in Psychology, 12*, 769459. [CrossRef]

Li, X., & Ye, Y. (2022). Fear of missing out and irrational procrastination in the mobile social media environment: A moderated mediation analysis. *Cyberpsychology, Behavior, and Social Networking, 25*(1), 59–65. [CrossRef]

Ma, X., Meng, D., Zhu, L., Xu, H., Guo, J., Yang, L., Yu, L., Fu, Y., & Mu, L. (2022). Bedtime procrastination predicts the prevalence and severity of poor sleep quality of Chinese undergraduate students. *Journal of American College Health, 70*(4), 1104–1111. [CrossRef]

Mayo, M. (2016). *The gender gap in feedback and self-perception*. Harvard Business Review. Available online: https://hbr.org/2016/08/the-gender-gap-in-feedback-and-self-perception (accessed on 30 August 2025).

Montag, C., Yang, H., & Elhai, J. D. (2021). On the psychology of TikTok use: A first glimpse from empirical findings. *Frontiers in Public Health, 9*, 641673. [CrossRef] [PubMed]

Muñoz-Rodríguez, J. M., Patino Alonso, C., Pessoa, T., & Martín-Lucas, J. (2023). Identity profile of young people experiencing a sense of risk on the internet: A data mining application of decision tree with CHAID algorithm. *Computers & Education, 197*, 104743. [CrossRef]

Naushad, K., Jamil, B., Khan, N. A., & Jadoon, M. (2025). Correlation between social media addiction and academic procrastination in medical students at public and private medical colleges at Peshawar. *Pakistan Journal of Medical Sciences, 41*(3), 837–842. [CrossRef] [PubMed]

Nicolaisen, M., & Thorsen, K. (2024). Gender differences in loneliness over time: A 15-year longitudinal study of men and women in the second part of life. *The International Journal of Aging and Human Development, 98*(1), 103–132. [CrossRef] [PubMed]

Niermann, H. C. M., & Scheres, A. (2014). The relation between procrastination and symptoms of attention-deficit hyperactivity disorder (ADHD) in undergraduate students: Role of procrastination in ADHD-related symptoms. *International Journal of Methods in Psychiatric Research, 23*(4), 411–421. [CrossRef]

Oberlo. (2023). *10 TikTok statistics you need to know in 2023*. Available online: https://www.shopify.com/blog/tiktok-statistics (accessed on 26 August 2025).

Pagan, R. (2020). Gender and age differences in loneliness: Evidence for people without and with disabilities. *International Journal of Environmental Research and Public Health, 17*(24), 9176. [CrossRef]

Pedrouzo, S., & Krynski, L. (2023). Hyperconnected: Children and adolescents on social media. The TikTok phenomenon. *Archivos Argentinos de Pediatria, 121*(4), e202202674. [CrossRef]

Pieh, C., Humer, E., Hoenigl, A., Schwab, J., Mayerhofer, D., Dale, R., & Haider, K. (2025). Smartphone screen time reduction improves mental health: A randomized controlled trial. *BMC Medicine, 23*(1), 107. [CrossRef]

Plackett, R., Blyth, A., & Schartau, P. (2023). The impact of social media use interventions on mental well-being: Systematic review. *Journal of Medical Internet Research, 25*, e44922. [CrossRef]

Pop, L. M., Iorga, M., & Iurcov, R. (2022). Body-esteem, self-esteem and loneliness among social media young users. *International Journal of Environmental Research and Public Health, 19*(9), 5064. [CrossRef]

Punzalan, M. J. P., Flores, N., Alvior, P. R., Villarubia, S., & Lazaro, B. L. (2024). Lost in the feed: Exploring the lived experiences of students on doomscrolling. *International Journal of Advanced Multidisciplinary Research and Studies, 4*(3), 378–385. [CrossRef]

Radtke, T., Apel, T., Schenkel, K., Keller, J., & von Lindern, E. (2021). Digital detox: An effective solution in the smartphone era? A systematic literature review. *Mobile Media & Communication, 10*(2), 190–215. [CrossRef]

Rasouli, A., Nejad-Ebrahim Soumee, Z., Tirgari Seraji, H., Ramzi, F., & Saed, O. (2025). The self-control bridge: Connecting social media use to academic procrastination. *Psychological Reports, under press*. [CrossRef]

Roberts, T.-A. (1991). Gender and the influence of evaluations on self-assessments in achievement settings. *Psychological Bulletin, 109*(2), 297–308. [CrossRef]

Rosenberg, M. (1965). *Society and the adolescent self-image*. Princeton University Press. [CrossRef]

Satici, S. A., Tekin, E. G., Deniz, M. E., & Satici, B. (2023). Doomscrolling scale: Its association with personality traits, psychological distress, social media use, and wellbeing. *Applied Research in Quality of Life, 18*, 833–847. [CrossRef]

Savoia, E., Harriman, N. W., Su, M., Cote, T., & Shortland, N. (2021). Adolescents' exposure to online risks: Gender disparities and vulnerabilities related to online behaviors. *International Journal of Environmental Research and Public Health, 18*(11), 5786. [CrossRef] [PubMed]

Seekis, V., & Kennedy, R. (2023). The impact of #beauty and #self-compassion tiktok videos on young women's appearance shame and anxiety, self-compassion, mood, and comparison processes. *Body Image, 45*, 117–125. [CrossRef] [PubMed]

Sipal, R. F., Karakaya, Y., & Hergul, N. (2011). I am online: What adolescents think about Internet and Internet use. *Procedia—Social and Behavioral Sciences, 30*, 2420–2426. [CrossRef]

Smith, T., & Short, A. (2022). Needs affordance as a key factor in likelihood of problematic social media use: Validation, latent Profile analysis and comparison of TikTok and Facebook problematic use measures. *Addictive Behaviors, 129*, 107259. [CrossRef]

Statista. (2023). *TikTok impact on mental health for U.S. users 2023.* Statista. Available online: https://www.statista.com/statistics/1409776/tiktom-us-opinions-mental-health-effects/ (accessed on 17 August 2025).

Statista. (2025). *Topic: Social media.* Statista. Available online: https://www.statista.com/topics/1164/social-networks/ (accessed on 17 August 2025).

Steel, P. (2010). Arousal, avoidant and decisional procrastinators: Do they exist? *Personality and Individual Differences, 48*(8), 926–934. [CrossRef]

Swart, J. (2021). Experiencing algorithms: How young people understand, feel about, and engage with algorithmic news selection on social media. *Social Media + Society, 7*(2), 20563051211008828. [CrossRef]

Vandenbroucke, J. P., Von Elm, E., Altman, D. G., Gøtzsche, P. C., Mulrow, C. D., Pocock, S. J., Poole, C., Schlesselman, J. J., Egger, M., & STROBE Initiative. (2007). Strengthening the Reporting of Observational Studies in Epidemiology (STROBE): Explanation and elaboration. *PLoS Medicine, 4*(10), e297. [CrossRef] [PubMed]

Wallaroomedia. (2024). *TikTok statistics—Everything you need to know.* Wallaroo Media. Available online: https://wallaroomedia.com/blog/tiktok-statistics/ (accessed on 17 August 2025).

Wang, Y., Jiang, W., & Wu, L. (2023). Association between age and loneliness in different residential type and gender groups: Evidence from China. *BMC Psychiatry, 23*(1), 43. [CrossRef] [PubMed]

World Medical Association. (2013). World Medical Association Declaration of Helsinki: Ethical principles for medical research involving human subjects. *JAMA, 310*(20), 2191. [CrossRef]

Wu, W., Zhang, J., & Jo, N. (2025). Fear of missing out and online social anxiety in university students: Mediation by irrational procrastination and media multitasking. *Behavioral Sciences, 15*(1), 84. [CrossRef]

Zacks, S., & Hen, M. (2018). Academic interventions for academic procrastination: A review of the literature. *Journal of Prevention & Intervention in the Community, 46*(2), 117–130. [CrossRef] [PubMed]

Zhou, X., Yang, F., Chen, Y., & Gao, Y. (2024). The correlation between mobile phone addiction and procrastination in students: A meta-analysis. *Journal of Affective Disorders, 346*, 317–328. [CrossRef]

European Journal of
Investigation in Health, Psychology and Education

MDPI

Review

Mediating and Moderating Mechanisms in the Relationship Between Social Media Use and Adolescent Aggression: A Scoping Review of Quantitative Evidence

Georgios Giannakopoulos [1,*] and Afroditi Prassou [2]

[1] Department of Child Psychiatry, School of Medicine, National and Kapodistrian University of Athens, 115 27 Athens, Greece
[2] 4th Directorate of Secondary Education of Athens, 171 21 Athens, Greece; aprassou@sch.gr
* Correspondence: ggiannak@med.uoa.gr

Abstract: Adolescents' pervasive use of social media has been increasingly linked to aggression, including cyberbullying and hostile online interactions. While this association is well documented, the psychological and contextual mechanisms that mediate or moderate it remain unclear. This scoping review maps quantitative evidence on mediators and moderators between social media use and aggression among adolescents. A comprehensive search using ProQuest's Summon platform was conducted across PsycINFO, Scopus, PubMed, and Web of Science, following the PRISMA 2020 guidelines. Eligible studies, published between January 2020 and March 2025, included adolescents aged 11–18 and reported at least one statistical mediation or moderation analysis. Forty-four studies from 19 countries (N > 90,000) were thematically synthesized. Key mediators included problematic use, moral disengagement, depression, attention-seeking, and risky digital behaviors. Moderators included gender, body satisfaction, cultural setting, school type, and family attachment. Most of the studies used structural equation modeling or PROCESS macro, although cross-sectional designs predominated. Limitations included reliance on self-reports and inconsistent social media measures. The findings suggest that social media–aggression links are indirect and shaped by emotional, cognitive, and ecological factors. Multi-level interventions targeting digital literacy, moral reasoning, and resilience are needed. This review was not registered and received no external funding.

Keywords: adolescent aggression; social media use; mediators; moderators

1. Introduction

In recent years, social media platforms such as Instagram, TikTok, and Snapchat have become central to adolescent life, shaping how youths communicate, present themselves, and navigate peer relationships (Ferreira et al., 2021; Martínez-Ferrer et al., 2021). Although these platforms offer opportunities for self-expression and social connection, a growing body of research has documented their association with various forms of aggression, including cyberbullying, hostile messaging, and digital retaliation (Colella et al., 2024; Ramírez et al., 2021). Given that over 90% of adolescents in many countries use social media daily (Soriano-Molina et al., 2025), understanding the psychosocial mechanisms linking digital engagement with aggression has become a public health priority.

While the correlation between social media use and adolescent aggression is well established (Madriaza et al., 2025), the recent scholarship has shifted toward identifying mediating and moderating variables that explain or condition this relationship. Mediators—such as problematic social media use, moral disengagement, or emotional vulnerabilities—shed light on how social media affects behavior (Gul et al., 2022; Liu et al., 2023; Tan, 2024). Moderators—including gender, age, cultural context, or body satisfaction—highlight the boundary conditions under which these effects vary (Geng et al., 2022; Jenkins et al., 2024; Wang et al., 2023). This focus aligns with ecological and developmental models that consider adolescent behavior as shaped by dynamic interactions between individual traits and social environments (Hernández et al., 2021; Shahnawaz et al., 2020).

Several theoretical frameworks have guided this line of research. The General Aggression Model (Allen et al., 2018) posits that situational inputs (e.g., cybervictimization) influence aggressive outcomes via internal affective and cognitive processes. For example, Colella et al. (2025) found that cybervictimization predicted cyberbullying through a serial mediation involving problematic social media use and moral disengagement. Their cross-national study of Italian and Spanish preadolescents revealed consistency in these pathways, suggesting cultural invariance in the psychosocial processes that escalate online conflict into aggression.

Other frameworks, such as the SPIN model (Status Pursuit in Narcissism) and social learning theory, emphasize the role of self-enhancement motives and peer feedback loops. Wang et al. (2023) reported that narcissism predicted both cyberbullying and online prosocial behavior via attention-seeking, but not impulsivity, indicating strategic rather than reactive aggression. Loneliness moderated this relationship, amplifying the effects of narcissistic traits on online behavior. Similarly, Geng et al. (2022) found that social comparison orientation led to the perpetration of cyberbullying and victimization via envy, particularly among adolescents with low body satisfaction—a pattern highlighting the emotional costs of appearance-based comparisons on social networking sites.

The cognitive dimension of aggression has also been explored through moral disengagement and identity-based mechanisms. Shahnawaz et al. (2020) found that sadism predicted cyber aggression, and that moral identity moderated this relationship in complex ways—acting both as a buffer and, paradoxically, as a predictor of aggression depending on internalization. Z. Zhang et al. (2022) demonstrated that dark triad traits (Machiavellianism, narcissism, psychopathy) predicted cyber aggression via moral disengagement, with gender differences moderating these pathways.

At the contextual level, parental communication, school climate, and cultural norms shape digital behavior. Achuthan et al. (2022) reported that both parental and adolescent gender moderated the influence of perceived parental control on cyber behavior. Chen et al. (2025) found that internet self-efficacy and online social capital mediated the relationship between cyberbullying and psychological distress, but only in public school students—indicating that educational context can moderate the efficacy of protective mechanisms. Jenkins et al. (2024) showed that students of color progressed more robustly through the cognitive stages of bystander intervention, even though actual intervention behavior was more common among White students—demonstrating racial variation in how moral cognition translates to action.

Despite these insights, the literature remains fragmented. Most studies have investigated mediators or moderators in isolation, often using cross-sectional designs and homogeneous samples. No systematic or scoping review to date has comprehensively examined the psychological and contextual mechanisms that mediate or moderate the relationship between social media use and adolescent aggression. This review addresses that gap by mapping the breadth and characteristics of 44 peer-reviewed quantitative studies published between 2020 and 2025.

This mapping is guided by three research questions: (1) What are the most consistently identified mediators and moderators linking social media use to adolescent aggression? (2) How do these mechanisms vary across demographic, cultural, or educational groups? (3) What methodological approaches are used to test these mechanisms, and what are their strengths and limitations? By addressing these questions, this review offers a structured empirical foundation for future theory development, prevention strategies, and culturally responsive interventions targeting aggression in digital adolescence.

2. Scoping Review Methodology

This scoping review was conducted in accordance with the PRISMA extension (PRISMA-ScR) to the PRISMA 2020 guidelines (Page et al., 2021; Tricco et al., 2018), which provides guidance for mapping the scope and nature of existing evidence. The review aimed to identify emerging patterns and themes in quantitative studies on mediating and moderating mechanisms, rather than to aggregate effect sizes or assess the strength of evidence, as would be expected in a formal systematic review. As a scoping review, the purpose was to map the existing literature, rather than to assess the strength or direction of effects across studies, as would be expected in a systematic review or meta-analysis. The goal was not to evaluate the evidence base for causal inference but to chart the types of mediating and moderating mechanisms examined, the methods used to test them, and how these variables were conceptually and statistically operationalized. This review thus offers breadth and thematic structure, rather than exhaustive or quantitative synthesis.

No formal protocol was prepared for this review. However, all methodological decisions were determined in advance and are reported transparently to ensure reproducibility. No amendments were made, as the review was not registered and no protocol was prepared. Although the review adhered to transparent and reproducible methods, the absence of a pre-registered protocol further aligns it with a scoping review framework, which emphasizes exploratory mapping of a research field.

The literature search was performed in March 2025 using ProQuest's Summon Discovery Service of the Library and Information Center at the National and Kapodistrian University of Athens. This platform aggregates results from a wide range of scholarly databases, including PsycINFO, Scopus, Web of Science, PubMed, and ScienceDirect, thus allowing for comprehensive coverage of interdisciplinary research in psychology, education, public health, and communication studies. The search covered studies published between January 2020 and March 2025.

The decision to restrict the review to studies published from 2020 onward was based on three key considerations: First, the digital media landscape has changed rapidly in recent years, with platforms such as TikTok and Instagram overtaking earlier networks in adolescent engagement patterns. Second, the period from 2020 to 2025 reflects a post-pandemic digital shift in youth behavior, marked by increased screen time, social isolation, and new forms of online interaction. Third, recent studies have increasingly adopted more sophisticated statistical models (e.g., PROCESS macro, structural equation modeling), allowing for a clearer and more theory-driven examination of mediating and moderating variables. This five-year window therefore captures the most methodologically and contextually relevant evidence available.

The following Boolean keyword combination was used: ("adolescent" OR "youth" OR "teenager") AND ("social media" OR "social networking" OR "Instagram" OR "TikTok" OR "Facebook") AND ("aggression" OR "cyberbullying" OR "hostility" OR "interpersonal violence") AND ("mediator" OR "moderator" OR "mediation" OR "moderation" OR "path analysis" OR "structural equation modeling" OR "PROCESS macro"). Filters were applied to restrict the results to peer-reviewed journal articles written in English and available in full text.

The inclusion criteria required that the studies (a) were published in English in peer-reviewed journals between 2020 and 2025; (b) focused on adolescents, typically aged 11 to 18; (c) employed quantitative methodologies; (d) examined aggression or related behavioral outcomes in connection to social media use; and (e) statistically tested at least one mediating or moderating variable. Studies were excluded if they addressed child or adult samples exclusively, employed qualitative or mixed-methods designs without quantifiable mediation or moderation analysis, or did not assess aggression-related outcomes. The authors screened all records for eligibility, including title/abstract screening and full-text review. No automation tools were used.

After the initial screening of 87 titles and abstracts, 81 articles were retained for full-text review. Of these, 37 were excluded for various reasons, including the absence of statistical mediation or moderation testing, irrelevant outcome variables, qualitative design, or age groups outside the adolescent range. Ultimately, 44 studies met all of the inclusion criteria and were included in the synthesis. The selection process is illustrated in a PRISMA-compliant flow diagram (Figure 1).

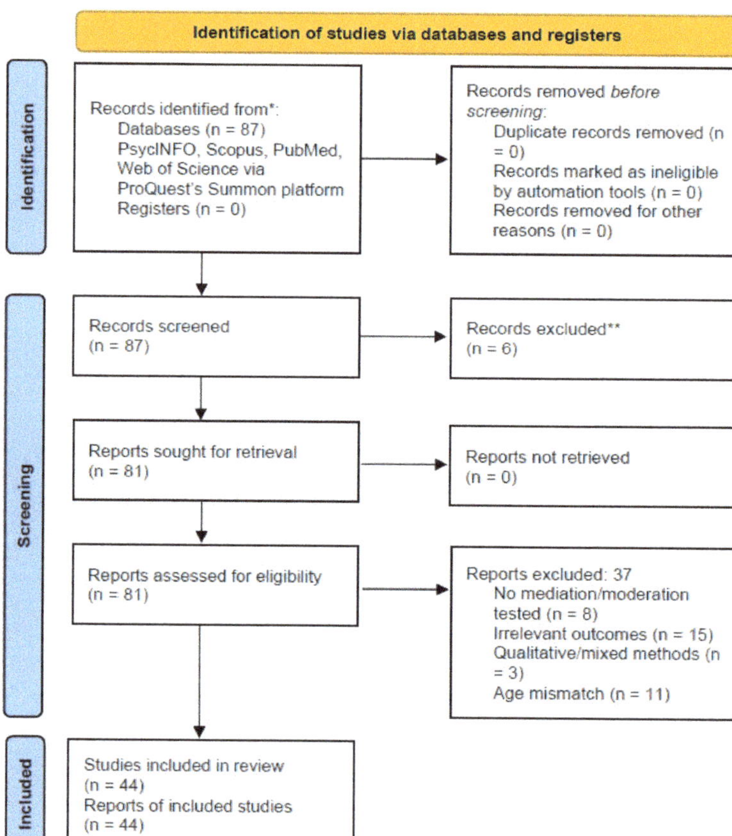

Figure 1. PRISMA flow diagram depicting the study selection process. * The total number across all databases/registers is reported. ** No automation tools were used for record exclusion.

The authors extracted data from all included studies using a standardized coding form. No automation tools were used, and no additional data were obtained from the study investigators. For each included study, the following variables were recorded: publication year, country of origin, sample size and characteristics, research design, type of aggression assessed (e.g., cyberbullying, digital dating abuse), social media constructs investigated (e.g., problematic use, exposure, communication behavior), mediators and moderators tested, statistical models employed (e.g., SEM, PROCESS macro), and key findings related to both direct and indirect effects.

Analytical Framework

To ensure consistency in data synthesis, a structured analytical framework was applied. Each included study was reviewed for (a) type and definition of aggression outcome, (b) operationalization of social media use, (c) mediating and/or moderating variables tested, (d) statistical model employed (e.g., SEM, PROCESS macro), and (e) sample characteristics, including age, gender, and cultural context. Mediators and moderators were coded based on thematic categories derived from theory, as outlined below. Rather than evaluating effect sizes, the review focused on the presence, direction, and statistical significance of each mediational or moderational pathway. This framework enabled the identification of recurrent mechanisms and cross-study convergence.

Given the heterogeneity in study designs, measurement instruments, and conceptualizations of both social media use and aggression, a meta-analytic synthesis was deemed inappropriate. Instead, a narrative thematic synthesis was employed to identify converging patterns and recurring mechanisms across cultural, methodological, and theoretical contexts. No sensitivity analyses were conducted, as the review was based on narrative synthesis rather than quantitative meta-analysis. The studies were grouped according to the primary type of mediating or moderating variable that they examined—such as psychological traits, cognitive mechanisms, emotional vulnerabilities, or sociocultural factors. Particular attention was given to methodological quality, statistical modeling approaches (e.g., serial and moderated mediation), and model fit indices, where reported. All reported quantitative outcomes related to adolescent aggression—such as cyberbullying perpetration, cybervictimization, digital dating abuse, and online hostility—were included. When multiple outcomes or timepoints were reported, the primary outcome, as defined by the study authors, was extracted. No data were excluded based on measurement instruments or timing. No data transformation, imputation, or conversion procedures were applied. All extracted information was used as reported in the primary studies. Given the narrative nature of the synthesis, missing or incomplete summary statistics were not a limiting factor. Additional data were extracted on study characteristics such as publication year, country of origin, participant age and sample size, study design, variables related to social media use and aggression, mediators and moderators, and analytic approach.

The categorization of mediators and moderators was informed by psychological theory, particularly the General Aggression Model (Allen et al., 2018), ecological systems theory (Bronfenbrenner, 1999), and contemporary models of adolescent socio-emotional development. Mediators were grouped based on their theoretical role in behavioral regulation (e.g., problematic use), cognitive processing (e.g., moral disengagement), emotional vulnerability (e.g., depression), self-concept (e.g., identity clarity), and social context (e.g., school climate). Moderators were organized according to their level of influence—individual (e.g., gender), interpersonal (e.g., parent–child dynamics), or sociocultural (e.g., national or educational context)—in line with ecological systems theory. This framework provided a theoretically grounded structure for the thematic synthesis.

Funding sources and conflicts of interest were not consistently reported and were therefore excluded from data extraction. When information was unclear or missing, the best available interpretation of the text was used; no study authors were contacted. Effect measures such as regression coefficients, odds ratios, or *p*-values were not systematically extracted, due to variability in reporting formats. Instead, the findings were synthesized based on the direction and presence of statistically significant mediation and moderation effects. Supplementary Table S1 summarizes the 44 included studies, highlighting study characteristics, tested mechanisms, and key findings.

Study quality was assessed by the authors through a narrative appraisal using the Mixed-Methods Appraisal Tool (MMAT; Hong et al., 2018), which evaluates five key domains: representativeness of participants, appropriateness of measurements, completeness of outcome data, adjustment for confounders, and nonresponse bias. No automation tools were used. Studies meeting at least four of the five criteria were considered to be of moderate-to-high quality. The majority of the studies (27 out of 44) met all five MMAT criteria, reflecting high methodological rigor. Common strengths included representative sampling, use of validated measurement instruments, and complete outcome reporting. However, approximately one in four studies partially addressed confounder adjustment, and one in five provided unclear reporting on nonresponse bias. Despite these limitations, the widespread use of sophisticated statistical modeling (e.g., SEM, PROCESS macro) across studies reinforces the reliability of the reported mediation and moderation effects.

The MMAT framework captured the completeness of outcome reporting at the study level; however, no formal assessment of reporting bias across the synthesis (e.g., publication bias or selective outcome reporting) was conducted. Funnel plot analysis and statistical tests were not applicable due to the narrative nature of the synthesis. Similarly, no formal assessment of certainty in the body of evidence was performed. While study-level quality was evaluated using the MMAT, frameworks such as GRADE were not applied to assess the overall confidence in outcome-level conclusions. The full MMAT results are presented in Supplementary Table S2.

3. Results

This scoping review mapped findings from 44 peer-reviewed quantitative studies conducted between 2020 and 2025, comprising data from over 90,000 adolescents across 19 countries. Although the studies varied in their design, sample composition, and conceptual frameworks, there was a high degree of convergence regarding the mediating and moderating mechanisms linking social media use to adolescent aggression. Most of the studies employed cross-sectional designs (n = 42), while only two utilized longitudinal or experimental methodologies. Structural equation modeling and PROCESS-based mediation/moderation analyses were the most frequently used analytic strategies. Thematic synthesis yielded five primary categories of mediators and four thematic groups of moderators, as outlined below.

It is important to emphasize that this is a scoping review, not a systematic review or meta-analysis. Therefore, the findings are not reported as standardized effect sizes or pooled estimates. Instead, the studies are grouped thematically based on common mechanisms and pathways to identify what has been studied, how often, and with what methodological approaches. This allows us to describe the landscape of existing evidence and identify theoretical and empirical gaps, which is consistent with the aims of scoping reviews.

3.1. Mediating Variables

The following categories of mediators were derived from an iterative thematic analysis informed by theory. Behavioral, cognitive, emotional, identity-related, and contextual domains were identified based on their alignment with ecological and psychosocial models of adolescent development and aggression. These categories reflect not only the nature of the variables but also their proposed functional role in linking social media use to aggressive outcomes.

3.1.1. Problematic Social Media Use

A consistent body of evidence identified problematic social media use as a robust mediator between digital engagement and aggression. Studies conceptualized this construct as a pattern of compulsive, emotionally dysregulated, or maladaptive engagement with social networking platforms. Colella et al. (2024, 2025) demonstrated that cybervictimization increased the likelihood of cyberbullying perpetration through sequential mediation by problematic social media use and moral disengagement. Similarly, Peprah et al. (2024) found that problematic use partially mediated the relationship between cybervictimization and psychosomatic complaints, accounting for approximately 12 percent of the total effect.

3.1.2. Moral Disengagement

Moral disengagement emerged as a key cognitive mediator across multiple studies, particularly those conducted in Italy, China, and Malaysia. In the work of Colella et al. (2025) and Piccardi et al. (2023), moral disengagement was found to mediate the relationship between problematic media use and cyberbullying. Tan (2024) employed a serial mediation model and demonstrated that false self-presentation led to increased moral disengagement, which, in turn, predicted cyber aggression and eventual social withdrawal. Z. Zhang et al. (2022) showed that moral disengagement mediated the link between dark triad personality traits and cyber aggression, with gender moderating these effects, particularly among female adolescents.

3.1.3. Emotional and Psychological Vulnerability

Numerous studies highlighted emotional vulnerabilities—such as depression, anxiety, attention-seeking, and distress—as mediating mechanisms. Wang et al. (2023) reported that attention-seeking behavior mediated the association between narcissism and both cyberbullying and prosocial online behaviors. Liu et al. (2023) identified depression as a mediating factor between cybervictimization and non-suicidal self-injury. Kim et al. (2024) added that loneliness and peer exclusion mediated the link between social media conflict and cybervictimization.

In addition to emotional distress, sleep quality also appears to mediate the relationship between problematic social media use and aggression. Lin et al. (2024) demonstrated that social media addiction predicted nighttime social media use and poorer sleep quality, which, in turn, led to greater aggression among early adolescents, suggesting that disrupted sleep may act as both a consequence of digital overuse and a driver of maladaptive behavior.

In the Turkish context, Doğrusever and Bilgin (2025) identified hostility and depression as serial mediators between low family social support and problematic internet use. Gul et al. (2022) provided further nuance, showing that psychiatric symptoms like somatization, hostility, and paranoid ideation increased smartphone overuse, while fear of missing out was linked specifically to anxiety and male gender, but not to depression or hostility.

3.1.4. Self-Concept, Identity, and Resilience

Several studies examined how self-related processes moderated or mediated the link between digital experiences and aggression. Kaakinen et al. (2021) found that risky online communication behaviors mediated the relationship between dating app use and various forms of victimization. Kee et al. (2024) demonstrated that psychological distress, including anxiety and emotional exhaustion, mediated the path from cyberbullying to suicidal ideation. Q. Pan et al. (2024) found that self-concept clarity and self-esteem jointly shaped adolescents' emotional sensitivity to problematic social media use. Y. Pan et al. (2024) showed that narcissism and self-control mediated the relationship between game addiction and aggression, with narcissism accounting for nearly half of the total effect. Bakan Kıraç et al. (2024) identified psychological resilience as a full mediator between internet addiction and anger control. Tamarit et al. (2021) added that sexting and body self-esteem mediated the link between internet addiction and sexual online victimization.

3.1.5. Cognitive and Social Processes

Cognitive appraisal and social learning mechanisms also emerged as explanatory pathways. Geng et al. (2022) identified envy on social media as a mediator between social comparison and both cyberbullying perpetration and victimization. Chen et al. (2025) reported that internet self-efficacy and online social capital mediated the relationship between victimization and mental health, although the latter was significant only among public school students. Maurya et al. (2023) demonstrated that parental communication and self-efficacy jointly mediated the effect of cybervictimization on depression. Hernández et al. (2021) linked personality traits such as narcissism and disinhibition to sexting and online grooming victimization. Mardianto et al. (2023) highlighted prejudice as a mediator between perceived threat, school climate, and cyber aggression. Reed et al. (2021) connected stereotypical gender beliefs to digital dating abuse via cognitive scripts regarding relational norms. Virat et al. (2024) emphasized societal mattering as a mediator between attitudinal disengagement and delinquent intent.

3.1.6. Environmental and Sociocultural Stressors

Laeheem (2024) found that, in Thailand's deep south, negative upbringing and exposure to violence predicted cyberbullying, with emotional traits like frustration and paranoia mediating the relationship. Marinoni et al. (2024) showed that time spent online during the COVID-19 pandemic mediated the effects of social media use on cyberbullying, with gender moderating this relationship. Yusuf et al. (2021) reported that internet exposure was a stronger predictor of aggression–victimization than family or peer attachment in Malaysia. Ramírez et al. (2021) found that sleep deprivation mediated the effect of weekday screen time on academic performance.

3.2. *Moderating Variables*

Moderators were organized into individual-level (e.g., gender, personality traits), interpersonal-level (e.g., parental relationships), and sociocultural-level (e.g., school type, national context) domains. This structure reflects an ecological framework emphasizing the multiple contexts that shape adolescent digital behavior.

3.2.1. Gender and Age

Gender emerged as a frequently tested moderator. Achuthan et al. (2022) found that parental and adolescent gender both moderated the link between parental control and adolescent behavior. Martínez-Ferrer et al. (2021) demonstrated that boys were more likely to cyberbully when controlling for problematic use. Aljasir and Alsebaei (2022) observed age and gender interactions in cybervictimization patterns, while Cebollero-Salinas et al. (2022) found age-related variation in the impact of cybergossip. Moreover, Alsebaei and Aljasir (2024) reported that parental demographic factors, including gender and education level, moderated the effectiveness of different mediation strategies on adolescent cyberbullying and cybervictimization, with technical mediation showing stronger effects among more educated parents.

3.2.2. Loneliness and Body Satisfaction

Wang et al. (2023) found that loneliness amplified the relationship between narcissism and attention-seeking, intensifying the pathway to aggression. Geng et al. (2022) showed that body satisfaction buffered the envy pathway between social comparison and cyber aggression.

3.2.3. Cultural and Contextual Moderators

Colella et al. (2025) confirmed model invariance across Italy and Spain. Chen et al. (2025) found that the school type moderated the buffering effect of online social capital. Achuthan et al. (2022) noted cultural differences between Indian and Singaporean adolescents in cyber conduct. Jenkins et al. (2024) identified racial differences in bystander intervention behavior in U.S. students. Alsebaei and Aljasir (2024), focusing on adolescents in Saudi Arabia, found that parental mediation strategies varied in effectiveness depending on cultural norms and parental education, underscoring the significance of sociocultural context in shaping digital parenting outcomes.

3.2.4. Psychological Traits and Parent–Child Relationships

Shahnawaz et al. (2020) showed that moral internalization moderated the effect of sadism on aggression. Qiu et al. (2024) found that empathy attenuated the effect of hostile attribution bias on online trolling. Strickland et al. (2023) revealed that parent–child closeness buffered the effect of cyber dating abuse on anxiety and depression. In a related study, Alsebaei and Aljasir (2024) found that parental mediation strategies—particularly technical and restrictive approaches—were more effective in reducing cyberbullying behaviors when combined with higher levels of parental education and digital awareness, highlighting the moderating role of family-level factors. Y. Zhang et al. (2021) highlighted that belief in negotiable fate and strong parental relationships jointly buffered the effect of psychological distress on cyber aggression during environmental crises.

4. Discussion

This scoping review mapped the findings from 44 peer-reviewed quantitative studies published between 2020 and 2025, with the aim of identifying mediating and moderating mechanisms in the relationship between social media use and adolescent aggression. The analysis revealed a multidimensional network of behavioral, cognitive, emotional, and contextual pathways that link digital engagement to aggressive outcomes. The results underscore that social media is not inherently conducive to aggression; rather, it is the convergence of individual vulnerabilities and environmental conditions that determines its psychological effects.

This review does not aim to aggregate or compare effect sizes across studies but, rather, to map how different psychological and contextual factors operate as mechanisms. Each mediating or moderating factor was analyzed in relation to its theoretical significance, frequency of appearance, and methodological treatment across studies. For example, emotional variables such as depression or attention-seeking were not only frequent but also embedded in multivariate models that link internal states to digital aggression. Likewise, cultural and environmental moderators, including school type and parental education, were often tested using subgroup or interaction analyses, reflecting increased attention to ecological specificity. Although most of the studies were cross-sectional, their cumulative design choices revealed a pattern of conceptual alignment with ecological and psychosocial frameworks.

The thematic convergence was strongest for mediators like problematic social media use and moral disengagement, but less consistency was observed in identity-related variables such as self-concept or narcissism. For example, some studies (Y. Pan et al., 2024) framed narcissism as a vulnerability, while others (Wang et al., 2023) linked it to strategic social navigation. Similarly, contextual mediators such as online self-efficacy (Chen et al., 2025) were shown to be protective only under specific educational settings, highlighting the role of the institutional environment as both a moderator and mediator. These divergences underscore the complex and sometimes contradictory ways in which psychological traits operate in digital spaces.

Problematic social media use emerged as the most recurrent and consistent mediator, often serving as the initial link in a chain of adverse psychological outcomes. Studies from both Western and Asian contexts, including those by Colella et al. (2024, 2025) and Peprah et al. (2024), showed that compulsive or dysregulated media use not only contributed directly to cyber aggression but also initiated subsequent mediational processes involving moral disengagement and psychosomatic distress. These findings align closely with the General Aggression Model (Allen et al., 2018), which posits that situational inputs such as cybervictimization influence behavior through internal states, including affect and cognition. In this context, problematic social media use acts as both a behavioral expression of distress and a vehicle through which adolescents become more exposed to risk-laden peer interactions and harmful content.

Moral disengagement was also a salient mechanism, appearing frequently in studies conducted across culturally diverse settings. It consistently mediated the relationship between problematic media use and aggression, often functioning as a cognitive rationalization process. Studies by Piccardi et al. (2023), Tan (2024), and Z. Zhang et al. (2022) emphasized how moral disengagement interacts with broader constructs such as self-presentation, emotional regulation, and personality traits. These findings suggest that cyber aggression is often not simply impulsive but may be framed by adolescents as morally excusable or socially justified, particularly in environments where accountability is attenuated.

In terms of emotional mechanisms, several pathways were identified that link psychological vulnerability to aggression through social media use. Attention-seeking (Wang et al., 2023), depression (Liu et al., 2023), and perceived social exclusion (Kim et al., 2024) were key mediators. Emotional dysregulation emerged as a recurring theme, particularly in the sequential pathways identified by Doğrusever and Bilgin (2025), where hostility and depression jointly mediated the effect of family support deficits on problematic internet use. In a related finding, Lin et al. (2024) demonstrated that sleep disturbance—mediated by nighttime social media use—served as a physiological pathway linking social media addiction to adolescent aggression, suggesting that behavioral dysregulation may be reinforced by impaired rest and recovery cycles. These findings reinforce developmental models of adolescence as a period of emotional volatility, and they provide empirical support for models that link social media engagement to emotional compensation strategies that may inadvertently increase the risk of aggression.

Beyond emotional factors, studies also illuminated the role of self-concept clarity, identity formation, and digital resilience. Q. Pan et al. (2024) showed that fragmented self-concept increased vulnerability to negative online interactions, while Y. Pan et al. (2024) highlighted the dual mediating role of narcissism and self-control in the link between gaming and aggression. Taken together, these findings suggest that digital aggression is embedded within larger processes of adolescent identity construction, especially in contexts where social validation and peer approval are increasingly pursued online.

The review also identified several sociocultural and environmental stressors that contribute to aggressive digital behavior. Laeheem (2024) linked negative upbringing and exposure to violence in politically unstable regions to cyberbullying, with emotional traits mediating the pathway. Yusuf et al. (2021) highlighted the predominance of internet exposure over familial attachments in predicting cyber aggression among Malaysian youths, while Marinoni et al. (2024) showed that pandemic-related increases in screen time mediated the effects of social media and gaming use on online aggression. These findings underscore that digital aggression cannot be fully understood without considering structural inequalities, environmental adversity, and broader social disruptions.

Moderating variables further nuanced the interpretation of these mediational pathways. Gender consistently shaped the strength and direction of the associations, as shown by Achuthan et al. (2022) and Martínez-Ferrer et al. (2021), although some studies challenged conventional gender patterns by highlighting interaction effects with personality traits (Shahnawaz et al., 2020). Other moderators included age, body satisfaction, and school type (Chen et al., 2025; Geng et al., 2022), as well as parent–child closeness (Strickland et al., 2023), parental education level (Alsebaei & Aljasir, 2024), and belief in negotiable fate (Y. Zhang et al., 2021). These moderators suggest that aggression outcomes are shaped not only by what adolescents experience but also by who they are, where they are, and how they interpret these experiences.

This review offers several key contributions. First, it establishes that the relationship between social media use and adolescent aggression is not direct but structured by a constellation of mediating and moderating factors. Second, it underscores the need for interventions that address not only behavioral regulation but also emotional, cognitive, and contextual dimensions. Programs that promote empathy, self-concept clarity, digital literacy, and moral reasoning may prove especially effective. Third, this review highlights the importance of tailoring prevention strategies to demographic and cultural contexts. For instance, fostering online social capital in under-resourced school settings or enhancing parental communication in collectivist cultures may yield distinct benefits.

Finally, these findings challenge the tendency to pathologize adolescent media use in blanket terms. Rather than viewing youths as passive recipients of digital harm, several studies in this review suggest that they are active agents navigating complex social ecosystems, sometimes with resilience and strategy. Future research should expand on this agency-oriented perspective by adopting longitudinal and mixed-methods designs, leveraging ecological models, and incorporating real-time behavioral metrics.

In conclusion, this review demonstrates that adolescent aggression in digital contexts emerges from the interactions between psychological vulnerabilities, cognitive frameworks, and environmental constraints. These insights call for multi-level, developmentally informed, and culturally sensitive approaches to prevention and intervention in an era where digital experiences increasingly shape adolescent development.

Limitations

This scoping review has several limitations. First, the search was restricted to English-language, peer-reviewed journal articles, which may have excluded relevant studies published in other languages or grey literature sources. Second, most of the included studies employed cross-sectional designs and self-report measures, limiting causal inference and introducing potential biases such as shared method variance. Third, variability in the measurement of key constructs—such as aggression and problematic social media use—made direct comparisons between studies difficult. Fourth, the narrative synthesis approach did not include effect size extraction or formal assessment of publication bias. Lastly, although a structured coding process was used, the review was conducted by a single author team without independent double screening or interrater reliability checks, which may have introduced interpretive bias.

5. Conclusions

This scoping review synthesized findings from 44 quantitative studies examining the mediating and moderating mechanisms between social media use and adolescent aggression. Rather than a direct relationship, the evidence reveals that digital aggression is shaped by a complex web of behavioral, cognitive, emotional, and contextual factors. Problematic social media use and moral disengagement were the most consistently identified mediators, while moderators such as gender, school type, and family attachment influenced the strength and direction of the effects. These findings underscore the importance of multi-level, theory-informed interventions that enhance digital resilience and psychosocial skills. Future research should prioritize longitudinal and mixed-methods designs to capture developmental trajectories and contextual nuance.

Supplementary Materials: The following supporting information can be downloaded at https://www.mdpi.com/article/10.3390/ejihpe15060098/s1: Table S1: Summary of included studies: mediators, moderators, and key findings; Table S2: Study quality assessment using the Mixed-Methods Appraisal Tool (MMAT); PRISMA-ScR checklist.

Author Contributions: Conceptualization, G.G. and A.P.; methodology, G.G.; software, G.G.; validation, G.G. and A.P.; formal analysis, G.G. and A.P.; investigation, G.G. and A.P.; resources, G.G.; data curation, G.G. and A.P.; writing—original draft preparation, G.G.; writing—review and editing, G.G. and A.P.; visualization, G.G.; supervision, G.G. All authors have read and agreed to the published version of the manuscript.

Funding: This research received no external funding.

Data Availability Statement: All data analyzed in this review were extracted from published studies and are summarized in the main manuscript and Supplementary Materials. No new datasets were generated or analyzed during the current study. Additional information is available from the corresponding author upon reasonable request.

Conflicts of Interest: The authors declare no conflicts of interest.

Abbreviations

The following abbreviations are used in this manuscript:

MMAT	Mixed-Methods Appraisal Tool
SEM	Structural equation modeling

References

Achuthan, K., Muthupalani, S., Kolil, V. K., & Madathil, K. C. (2022). Theoretical perspectives of parental influence on adolescent cyber behaviour: A bi-national Instagram-based study. *Heliyon*, *8*(11), e11813. [CrossRef] [PubMed]

Aljasir, S. A., & Alsebaei, M. O. (2022). Cyberbullying and cybervictimization on digital media platforms: The role of demographic variables and parental mediation strategies. *Humanities and Social Sciences Communications*, *9*(1), 320. [CrossRef]

Allen, J. J., Anderson, C. A., & Bushman, B. J. (2018). The General Aggression Model. *Current Opinion in Psychology*, *19*, 75–80. [CrossRef]

Alsebaei, M.-O., & Aljasir, S. A. (2024). Parenting in the digital age: Mediation strategies as a preventive factor against cyberbullying on social media among saudi parents. *Communication & Society*, *37*(4), 143–162.

Bakan Kıraç, İ., Sahmurova, A., Duradoni, M., Guazzini, A., & Gursesli, M. C. (2024). The shield of resilience: Mediating the effects of internet addiction on adolescent anger control. *Advances in Public Health*, *2024*(1), 5519519. [CrossRef]

Bronfenbrenner, U. (1999). Environments in developmental perspective: Theoretical and operational models. In *Measuring environment across the life span: Emerging methods and concepts* (pp. 3–28). American Psychological Association. [CrossRef]

Cebollero-Salinas, A., Orejudo, S., Cano-Escoriaza, J., & Íñiguez-Berrozpe, T. (2022). Cybergossip and problematic internet use in cyberaggression and cybervictimisation among adolescents. *Computers in Human Behavior*, *131*, 107230. [CrossRef]

Chen, Q., Guo, S., & Chan, K. L. (2025). Exploring the relationships among online social capital, internet self-efficacy, mental health, and cyberbully-victim roles in adolescents: A structural equation model. *Frontiers in Psychiatry*, *16*, 1427655. [CrossRef]

Colella, G. M., Palermiti, A. L., Bartolo, M. G., Servidio, R. C., & Costabile, A. (2024). Problematic social media use, retaliation, and moral disengagement in cyberbullying and cybervictimization among italian preadolescents: A moderated mediation model. *International Journal of Bullying Prevention*. [CrossRef]

Colella, G. M., Servidio, R. C., Palermiti, A. L., Bartolo, M. G., García-Carrera, P., Ortega-Ruiz, R., & Romera, E. M. (2025). Cyberbullying perpetration and socio-behavioral correlates in italian and spanish preadolescents: A cross-national study and serial mediation analysis. *International Journal of Environmental Research and Public Health*, *22*(3), 389. [CrossRef]

Doğrusever, C., & Bilgin, M. (2025). From family social support to problematic internet use: A serial mediation model of hostility and depression. *BMC Psychology*, *13*(1), 178. [CrossRef]

Ferreira, P. d. C., Veiga Simão, A. M., Pereira, N. S., Paulino, P., & Oliveira, S. (2021). Online verbal aggression, social relationships, and self-efficacy beliefs. *New Media & Society*, *23*(5), 960–981. [CrossRef]

Geng, J., Wang, Y., Wang, H., Wang, P., & Lei, L. (2022). Social comparison orientation and cyberbullying perpetration and victimization: Roles of envy on social networking sites and body satisfaction. *Journal of Interpersonal Violence*, *37*(17–18), NP16060–NP16083. [CrossRef] [PubMed]

Gul, H., Firat, S., Sertcelik, M., Gul, A., Gurel, Y., & Kilic, B. G. (2022). Effects of psychiatric symptoms, age, and gender on fear of missing out (FoMO) and problematic smartphone use: A path analysis with clinical-based adolescent sample. *Indian Journal of Psychiatry*, *64*(3), 289–294. [CrossRef] [PubMed]

Hernández, M. P., Schoeps, K., Maganto, C., & Montoya-Castilla, I. (2021). The risk of sexual-erotic online behavior in adolescents—Which personality factors predict sexting and grooming victimization? *Computers in Human Behavior*, *114*, 106569. [CrossRef]

Hong, Q. N., Fàbregues, S., Bartlett, G., Boardman, F., Cargo, M., Dagenais, P., Gagnon, M.-P., Griffiths, F., Nicolau, B., O'Cathain, A., Rousseau, M.-C., Vedel, I., & Pluye, P. (2018). The Mixed Methods Appraisal Tool (MMAT) version 2018 for information professionals and researchers. *Education for Information*, *34*(4), 285–291. [CrossRef]

Jenkins, L. N., Fredrick, S. S., & King, J. a. (2024). Testing the bystander intervention model in cyberbullying across students of color and white students. *International Journal of Bullying Prevention*, *6*(4), 389–398. [CrossRef]

Kaakinen, M., Koivula, A., Savolainen, I., Sirola, A., Mikkola, M., Zych, I., Paek, H. J., & Oksanen, A. (2021). Online dating applications and risk of youth victimization: A lifestyle exposure perspective. *Aggressive Behavior*, *47*(5), 530–543. [CrossRef]

Kee, D. M. H., Anwar, A., & Vranjes, I. (2024). Cyberbullying victimization and suicide ideation: The mediating role of psychological distress among Malaysian youth. *Computers in Human Behavior*, *150*, 108000. [CrossRef]

Kim, S., Garthe, R., Hsieh, W.-J., & Hong, J. S. (2024). Problematic social media use and conflict, social stress, and cyber-victimization among early adolescents. *Child and Adolescent Social Work Journal*, *41*(2), 223–233. [CrossRef]

Laeheem, K. (2024). Causal factors contributing to youth cyberbullying in the deep south of Thailand. *Children*, *11*(7), 790. [CrossRef]

Lin, S., Longobardi, C., Gastaldi, F. G. M., & Fabris, M. A. (2024). Social media addiction and aggressive behaviors in early adolescents: The mediating role of nighttime social media use and sleep quality. *The Journal of Early Adolescence*, *44*(1), 41–58. [CrossRef]

Liu, S., Wu, W., Zou, H., Chen, Y., Xu, L., Zhang, W., Yu, C., & Zhen, S. (2023). Cybervictimization and non-suicidal self-injury among Chinese adolescents: The effect of depression and school connectedness. *Frontiers in Public Health*, *11*, 1091959. [CrossRef] [PubMed]

Madriaza, P., Hassan, G., Brouillette-Alarie, S., Mounchingam, A. N., Durocher-Corfa, L., Borokhovski, E., Pickup, D., & Paillé, S. (2025). Exposure to hate in online and traditional media: A systematic review and meta-analysis of the impact of this exposure on individuals and communities. *Campbell Systematic Reviews*, *21*(1), e70018. [CrossRef]

Mardianto, M., Hartati, N., Aulia, F., Fikry, Z., Utami, R. H., & Magistarina, E. (2023). Contribution threat perception, school climate and prejudice as mediator to student's cyber aggression. *Journal of Cybersecurity*, *9*(1), tyac017. [CrossRef]

Marinoni, C., Rizzo, M., & Zanetti, M. A. (2024). Social media, online gaming, and cyberbullying during the COVID-19 pandemic: The mediation effect of time spent online. *Adolescents*, *4*(2), 297–310. [CrossRef]

Martínez-Ferrer, B., León-Moreno, C., Suárez-Relinque, C., Del Moral-Arroyo, G., & Musitu-Ochoa, G. (2021). Cybervictimization, offline victimization, and cyberbullying: The mediating role of the problematic use of social networking sites in boys and girls. *Psychosocial Intervention*, *30*(3), 155–162. [CrossRef]

Maurya, C., Muhammad, T., Das, A., Fathah, A., & Dhillon, P. (2023). The role of self-efficacy and parental communication in the association between cyber victimization and depression among adolescents and young adults: A structural equation model. *BMC Psychiatry, 23*(1), 337. [CrossRef]

Page, M. J., McKenzie, J. E., Bossuyt, P. M., Boutron, I., Hoffmann, T. C., Mulrow, C. D., Shamseer, L., Tetzlaff, J. M., Akl, E. A., Brennan, S. E., Chou, R., Glanville, J., Grimshaw, J. M., Hróbjartsson, A., Lalu, M. M., Li, T., Loder, E. W., Mayo-Wilson, E., McDonald, S., ... McGuinness, L. A. (2021). The PRISMA 2020 statement: An updated guideline for reporting systematic reviews. *BMJ, 372*, n71. [CrossRef]

Pan, Q., Lan, M., Tan, C. Y., Tao, S., Liang, Q., & Law, N. (2024). Protective factors contributing to adolescents' multifaceted digital resilience for their wellbeing: A socio-ecological perspective. *Computers in Human Behavior, 155*, 108164. [CrossRef]

Pan, Y., Motevalli, S., & Yu, L. (2024). The relationship between game addiction and aggression among adolescents with mediating role of narcissism and self-control. *Iranian Journal of Psychiatry, 19*(3), 274–284. [CrossRef]

Peprah, P., Oduro, M. S., Atta-Osei, G., Addo, I. Y., Morgan, A. K., & Gyasi, R. M. (2024). Problematic social media use mediates the effect of cyberbullying victimisation on psychosomatic complaints in adolescents. *Scientific Reports, 14*(1), 9773. [CrossRef] [PubMed]

Piccardi, L., Burrai, J., Palmiero, M., Quaglieri, A., Lausi, G., Cordellieri, P., Fraschetti, A., Giannini, A. M., & Mari, E. (2023). A cross-sectional study of gender role adherence, moral disengagement mechanisms and online vulnerability in adolescents. *Heliyon, 9*(8), e18910. [CrossRef] [PubMed]

Qiu, Y., Sun, Q., Wu, B., & Li, F. (2024). Is high exposure to antisocial media content associated with increased participation in malicious online trolling? exploring the moderated mediation model of hostile attribution bias and empathy. *BMC Psychology, 12*(1), 401. [CrossRef] [PubMed]

Ramírez, S., Gana, S., Garcés, S., Zúñiga, T., Araya, R., & Gaete, J. (2021). Use of technology and its association with academic performance and life satisfaction among children and adolescents. *Frontiers in Psychiatry, 12*, 764054. [CrossRef]

Reed, L. A., Ward, L. M., Tolman, R. M., Lippman, J. R., & Seabrook, R. C. (2021). The association between stereotypical gender and dating beliefs and digital dating abuse perpetration in adolescent dating relationships. *Journal of Interpersonal Violence, 36*(9–10), NP5561–NP5585. [CrossRef]

Shahnawaz, M. G., Shagufta, N., & Rehman, U. (2020). Sadism and cyber aggression: Moral identity as a possible moderator. *Journal of Aggression, Maltreatment & Trauma, 29*(8), 969–983. [CrossRef]

Soriano-Molina, E., Limiñana-Gras, R. M., Patró-Hernández, R. M., & Rubio-Aparicio, M. (2025). The association between internet addiction and adolescents' mental health: A meta-analytic review. *Behavioral Sciences, 15*(2), 116. [CrossRef]

Strickland, M. L., Love, H., & Kimmes, J. (2023). The interaction between adolescent cyber dating abuse and parenting on mental health outcomes. *Journal of Child and Family Studies, 32*(3), 769–780. [CrossRef]

Tamarit, A., Schoeps, K., Peris-Hernández, M., & Montoya-Castilla, I. (2021). The impact of adolescent internet addiction on sexual online victimization: The mediating effects of sexting and body self-esteem. *International Journal of Environmental Research and Public Health, 18*(8), 4226. [CrossRef]

Tan, C. S. L. (2024). All by myself: Examining social media's effect on social withdrawal and the mediating roles of moral disengagement and cyberaggression. *European Journal of Marketing, 58*(2), 659–684. [CrossRef]

Tricco, A. C., Lillie, E., Zarin, W., O'Brien, K. K., Colquhoun, H., Levac, D., Moher, D., Peters, M. D. J., Horsley, T., Weeks, L., Hempel, S., Akl, E. A., Chang, C., McGowan, J., Stewart, L., Hartling, L., Aldcroft, A., Wilson, M. G., Garritty, C., ... Lewin, S. (2018). PRISMA Extension for Scoping Reviews (PRISMA-ScR): Checklist and Explanation. *Annals of Internal Medicine, 169*(7), 467–473. [CrossRef] [PubMed]

Virat, M., Flett, G., Massez, L., & Przygodzki-Lionet, N. (2024). Low sense of mattering in society and delinquency among young people: An initial investigation. *Criminal Behaviour and Mental Health, 34*(6), 494–509. [CrossRef] [PubMed]

Wang, Y., Hawk, S. T., Wong, N., & Zhang, Y. (2023). Lonely, impulsive, and seeking attention: Predictors of narcissistic adolescents' antisocial and prosocial behaviors on social media. *International Journal of Behavioral Development, 47*(6), 540–547. [CrossRef]

Yusuf, S., Mohamed Al-Majdhoub, F., Mubin, N. N., Chaniago, R. H., & Rahim Khan, F. (2021). Cyber aggression-victimization among Malaysians youth. *Asian Journal of University Education (AJUE), 7*(1), 240–260. [CrossRef]

Zhang, Y., Xu, C., Dai, H., & Jia, X. (2021). Psychological distress and adolescents' cyberbullying under floods and the COVID-19 pandemic: Parent–child relationships and negotiable fate as moderators. *International Journal of Environmental Research and Public Health, 18*(23), 12279. [CrossRef]

Zhang, Z., Bian, S., Zhao, H., & Qi, C. (2022). Dark triad and cyber aggression among Chinese adolescents during COVID-19: A moderated mediation model. *Frontiers in Psychology, 13*, 1011123. [CrossRef]

European Journal of
Investigation in Health, Psychology and Education

MDPI

Article

Association Between Social Networking Service Use and Body Image Among Elementary School Children in Japan

Asami Baba [1], Masumi Suzuki [2], Rikako Yoshitake [1], Yumiko Inose [3] and Naomi Omi [1,4,*]

1 Graduate School of Comprehensive Human Sciences, University of Tsukuba, Ibaraki 305-8574, Japan; s2330477@u.tsukuba.ac.jp (A.B.); s2230490@u.tsukuba.ac.jp (R.Y.)
2 Gakuen no Mori Compulsory Education School, Ibaraki 305-0816, Japan; suzuki.masumi@mail.ibk.ed.jp
3 Department of Health and Nutrition, Faculty of Human Sciences, Tokiwa University, Ibaraki 310-0911, Japan; y-inose@tokiwa-u.jp
4 Institute of Health and Sports Sciences, University of Tsukuba, Ibaraki 305-8574, Japan
* Correspondence: omi.naomi.gn@u.tsukuba.ac.jp

Abstract: The number of studies suggesting that social networking services (SNSs) use poses a risk to children's body image continue to expand, but most studies have focused on adolescents. The study aimed to examine the associations between SNS use and body image among elementary school children in Japan. This study examined the relationship between SNSs use and body size perception and preference, body size misperception, and ideal body image among 1261 preadolescents (611 boys and 650 girls), aged 8–12 years (mean age = 9.64; SD =1.15; 52% girls), separately by sex. Using hierarchical multivariate linear regression analyses and logistic regression analyses, we examined body image factors and SNS use as the dependent and independent variables, respectively. Findings indicate that children who use SNSs do not significantly differ from nonusers regarding body dissatisfaction. However, SNS use is positively associated with body size misperception in girls. Additionally, for boys and girls, SNS use seems to increase the likelihood of admiring the body image of media figures rather than friends or classmates. Understanding how SNS use influences body image remains important for promoting healthy development in children.

Keywords: body image; body size perception and preference; body size misperception; ideal body image; preadolescents; social networking services

1. Introduction

Media exposure has been linked to body image concerns among youth. Most studies have focused on exposure to mass media formats such as television programs, magazines, and advertisements. However, given the extensive SNS use by young adults (Duggan & Smith, 2013), it has become increasingly important to study the potential relationship between SNS use and body image concerns among young boys and girls. SNS use has been associated with problematic behaviors related to actual body image, such as excessive food restriction and investment in appearance (Mabe et al., 2014; Vandenbosch & Eggermont, 2016). In particular, social comparison use has been associated with higher levels of bulimic symptoms and eating disorders (Smith et al., 2013). Therefore, identifying associations with SNS use is critical in addressing issues related to body image.

1.1. SNS Use and Body Size Perception and Preference

Social networking services (SNSs) considerably influence body image. Increased SNS use has been linked to body image disturbances and eating disorders in youth and adults, with small to moderate effect sizes (Holl& & Tiggemann, 2016; Huang et al., 2021; Saiphoo & Vahedi, 2019; Zhang et al., 2021). Recent studies have also suggested that higher media dependence is associated with body image disturbances in adolescents (Karam et al., 2023). Moreover, SNSs addiction was found to be associated directly with eating disorders and indirectly with poor body image in adolescents and young adults (Mohsenpour et al., 2023). Additionally, heavy SNS use has been associated with body size perception and preference among Australian preadolescents (mean age = 12.76; Rodgers et al., 2020). Thus, SNS use is a factor that affects body size perception and preference and body image disturbance in young people. Forming a proper body image at an early age is crucial for long-term healthy body development. However, the effects of SNS use on body image disturbance extend beyond body size perception and preference.

1.2. SNS Use and Body Size Misperception

SNS use also seems to affect body size misperception. Body size misperception is the discrepancy between one's perceived weight and one's actual weight status and is the result of a perceptual disorder that does not accurately assess one's body size, combined with body dissatisfaction, including negative feelings and cognitions about one's body (Liechty, 2010; Hosseini & Padhy, 2023). A study of Korean middle and high school students found that SNS dependence contributed to increased body size misperception (Cho et al., 2024). While studies on SNS use and body size misperception remain limited, these distortions can have serious physical implications. Incorrect body size misperception can lead to greater body size perception and preference. Body size misperception may be associated with eating disorders, unhealthy weight control behaviors, and mental health issues, including depression (Hosseini & Padhy, 2023). In turn, this may lead to the belief that one is overweight or underweight despite having a normal weight, excessive weight loss concerns, and an increased risk of eating disorders (e.g., overeating and underrating). Conversely, improving body size misperception may reduce body size perception and preference and social comparison, fostering healthier eating and self-care behaviors. Further investigation into the relationship between SNS use and body size misperception is necessary.

1.3. SNS Use and Ideal Body Image

Furthermore, the rapid expansion of SNS use has reshaped the ideal body image (IBI) standards. In the 2000s, before SNSs became a dominant information source, appearance-related pressures were believed to stem from the following three main sources: family, peers, and traditional media. These pressures would cause adolescent girls to internalize a thin appearance as ideal and make social appearance comparisons, resulting in body dissatisfaction (Webb & Zimmer-Gembeck, 2014; Scully et al., 2023). Family and friends' dieting behavior could influence them (Dixon et al., 1996). Traditional media, including television and fashion magazines, promoted the desire for thinness in young women through their portrayal of thin models and celebrities (British Medical Association, 2000). However, in recent years, adolescent girls' main information sources have shifted from television to SNSs (Derenne & Beresin, 2018; Ministry of Internal Affairs and Communications, 2021). This suggests that the highly visual SNSs may influence the overestimation of body image, the fear of weight gain, and the obsession with body image, promoting eating disorders (Sharma & Vidal, 2023). Viewing appearance-focused content and negative online social comparisons on SNSs indicates increased body dissatisfaction (Dane & Bhatia, 2023). A study found that people are more likely to internalize a thin-ideal image when comparing their appearance with others of the same gender on SNSs than when comparing themselves to friends or with models on TV or in fashion magazines (Holl& & Tiggemann, 2016). This suggests that SNS-based body comparisons, rather than those involving close family or friends, may reinforce the desire to lose weight and reinforce restrictive eating. Consequently, for many youths, the IBI may be shaped by people on SNSs.

1.4. Differences Among Girls and Boys

The impact of SNS use on body image is particularly pronounced in girls. Compared to boys, girls use SNSs at higher rates (Common Sense, 2022) and face greater risks of body image disturbances (Neumark-Sztainer et al., 2018) compared to boys. Generally, appearance is more important in girls' peer relations than among boys (Vannatta et al., 2009), and girls are reported as more susceptible to interpersonal influences from parents and peers than boys (Shulman, 1993). Exposure to idealized body images on SNSs has been associated with lower body satisfaction in girls, likely because of social comparison processes (Bucchianeri et al., 2013). Additionally, earlier puberty onset in girls than in boys (Patton & Viner, 2007) may contribute to significant sex differences in early body image assessment. Recently, concerns have been raised about assessing body image in adolescent boys to capture key aspects of boys' body image (Hansson & Schmidt, 2025). Many studies confirm increased body size perception and preference in girls, whilst its prevalence and patterns in boys remain less clear.

However, recent trends indicate a rising prevalence of thinness among preadolescent boys in Japan (Ministry of Education, Culture, Sports, Science and Technology, 2024a). In Japan, 1.3% of boys aged 8–9 and 2.6% of those aged 10–12 are categorized as thin, compared to 1.6% and 2.8% of girls in the same age groups, respectively. Since 1977, the proportion of underweight girls has remained stable, whereas rates have increased among boys (Ministry of Education, Culture, Sports, Science and Technology, 2024a). Globally, adolescent boys also experience body dissatisfaction and eating disorders symptoms (Ricciardelli & McCabe, 2002) and frequently use SNSs (Common Sense, 2022). Additionally, preliminary reports suggest that body image issues are significant concerns for boys (Nagata et al., 2021; Pope et al., 2000b), and boys experience pressure to lose weight (Sato & Tsuchiya, 2010). Given that thinness and body size misperception are key risk factors for eating disorders (Miyazaki & Ogata, 2006), body image disturbances represent a significant public health concern in Japan. Furthermore, boys generally have more of the ideal of body muscularity compared to girls (Pope et al., 2000a; Ricciardelli & Yager, 2015). Even with the same thinness judgments, there may be differences between boys and girls in their ideals for body image. Therefore, efforts should focus on fostering a healthy body image before adolescence and education to prevent unhealthy dieting for both sexes.

1.5. Preadolescent Media Use

Although previous research has primarily focused on adults, relatively little attention has been given to preadolescents. Whilst substantial evidence links SNS use to body image disturbances and eating disorders (Holl& & Tiggemann, 2016; Huang et al., 2021; Rapee et al., 2019), studies have specifically examined relationships between SNS use and body image in preteen samples. However, although SNS use increases rapidly from age 12 onwards (Smahel et al., 2020), the number of preadolescent SNS users has surged globally. In Japan, 98.1% of schoolchildren in grades 4–6 (ages 9–12) use digital media, and 58% have reported using SNSs such as LINE (48%), TikTok (31%), Instagram (9%), and X (2%) (Mobile Society Research Institute, 2023). The average daily screentime for this age group is 167.7 min, with 41.4% of them having 3 or more hours of screentime daily (Japan Sports Agency, 2024). These findings suggest that a substantial proportion of Japanese children engage with SNSs before adolescence. Given the annual surge of screentime use yearly and the decreasing age of SNS users, SNSs now constitute a critical environment for children today. Because much of children's social and emotional development occurs online, SNSs exert a much greater influence. However, most children possess limited self-regulation skills and remain vulnerable to peer pressure, increasing their risk of the negative outcomes associated with SNSs (Mohsenpour et al., 2023).

Both boys and girls have reported body size perception and preference before preadolescence (Grogan, 2016). These patterns indicate that SNS use may contribute to body image disturbances even before adolescence. Therefore, examining how SNS use relates to body image, including sex differences, is essential for addressing these issues in preadolescents.

1.6. The Current Study

The relationship between SNS use and body image has been examined in adolescence but has not been tested in preadolescence. The study aimed to examine the associations between SNS use and body image among preadolescent girls and boys. Specifically, this study explores its relationship with body size perception and preference, body size misperception, and IBI.

According to previous research examining the association between SNS use and body size perception and preference in adolescents, SNS use is a factor that affects body size perception and preference. This study addresses the understudied area of SNS use and body image among preadolescent children. By providing a more detailed examination of body image and exploring sex differences, it represents an initial effort to bridge the gap in previous research. Even in preadolescents, it may be hypothesized that children who use SNSs more frequently will be more dissatisfied with their bodies than children who use SNSs less frequently (Hypothesis 1). Previous research also indicates that incorrect body size perception may lead to greater body size perception and preference. It is thus hypothesized that children who use SNSs will have a greater size misperception towards body image (Hypothesis 2). Furthermore, because it could be predicted that IBI is also changing with the spread of SNSs, it could be hypothesized that children who use SNSs will have an IBI of media figures instead of their friends and classmates (Hypothesis 3).

2. Materials and Methods

2.1. Participants and Procedures

This cross-sectional study included 1261 third- to sixth-grade preadolescents (611 boys, 650 girls) aged 8–12 years (mean age = 9.64; SD = 1.15, 52% girls) from two urban public schools in Japan. Data were collected using a self-reported questionnaire. To obtain approval, school principals were first contacted and provided with information on the study's aims and questionnaire content. Once they granted permission, class teachers then distributed documents to parents stating the study's purpose, methods, data protection measures, results dissemination, and voluntary participation, asking for written consent for their schoolchild's participation. Finally, participants gave digital consent by selecting either "I agree to participate" or "I do not agree to participate." The privacy rights of participants have been observed and informed consent was obtained from the parents and preadolescents. If they chose not to participate, participants' decisions were acknowledged and the questionnaire was then terminated. Additionally, participants could also withdraw at any time by closing the browser without their answers being recorded.

The questionnaire was administered via self-report Google Forms on tablets. Data collection occurred during school hours and in a group setting with staff members present between May and June 2024. The questionnaire took approximately 20 min to complete. To ensure clarity and consistency, staff members explained the intent and wording of the questions to participants. The questionnaire avoided technical terms and unfamiliar kanji characters. The school principal, classroom teacher, and nutrition teacher reviewed the questionnaire. Moreover, to avoid missing data, incorrectly completed questionnaires, and entry mistakes, all questions were set as mandatory, and all answers were selected from predefined options. Before full administration, all measures were tested with a small sample of preadolescents and were assessed to be understandable for this age group.

A total of 1525 schoolchildren participated in the survey, but 264 were excluded because of nonresponses to the questions. Hence, the 1261 children who provided valid responses (valid response rate: 82.7%) were included in the analysis. Each dataset was assigned to a unique ID corresponding to demographic characteristics and questionnaire responses. Identifying details were then discarded after the dataset was created and managed using the ID. Participants' height and weight information were compared to the national average (Ministry of Education, Culture, Sports, Science and Technology, 2024a) using Student's *t*-test. No significant differences in height and weight were found for either sex.

This study received ethical approval from the Ethics Committee of the Faculty at the university.

2.2. General Situation of the Study Area

This study area covered the Kenkyu-gakuen district of Tsukuba City, Ibaraki Prefecture, Japan, in southwestern Ibaraki, approximately 50 km southwest of the prefectural capital and 50 km northeast of Tokyo (Tsukuba City Official Website, 2025). Its population is 241,656 (Ibaraki Prefectural Government, 2022), and it has the highest population growth rate in Japan (2.3%) (Ministry of Internal Affairs and Communications, 2021). The second school was in Fukuoka City, the capital and largest city of Fukuoka Prefecture, located in the western Kyushu region (Fukuoka City Official Website, 2025a). Fukuoka City has a population of 1,658,999 and 890,695 households (Fukuoka City Official Website, 2025b). Among ordinance-designated cities, it ranks first in the population growth rate and the proportion of young people in their teens and twenties (Fukuoka City Official Website, 2025a).

Both schools have well-developed information and communication technology (ICT)-based educational systems that incorporate tablet-based learning, digital textbooks, and online exchanges.

2.3. Measures

2.3.1. Demographic Characteristics

Participants' age, sex, standing height, and weight were recorded. Age, sex, height, and weight measurements were obtained from health checkups conducted in April 2024, and the obesity index (Japan Society of School Health, 2015) was calculated using these values. Additionally, physical fitness scores were collected from the results of the school's new physical fitness test, administered during the same period. Overweight and underweight were determined using the measured height and weight.

In Japan, the percentage of overweight (POW), a metric more commonly used for children than BMI-for-age percentile, is calculated based on the measured weight and standard weight-for-height as follows: POW (%) = 100 × (measured weight − standard weight-for-height)/standard weight-for-height. The standard weight-for-height was defined based on age- and sex-specific weight-for-height data from the 2024 Annual Report of School Health Statistics from the Ministry of Education, Culture, Sports, Science and Technology (2024a). Japanese standard weight was calculated using an equation derived from height and weight distributions at each age (Murata & Ito, 2003). The normal POW range for school-age children was between −20% and 20%. POWs of between −<30% and −<20%, and −≤ 30% were defined as moderate and severe thinness, respectively. POWs of between ≥20% and <30%, between ≥30% and <50%, and ≥50% were defined as mild, moderate, and severe obesity, respectively.

2.3.2. SNS Use

The purpose of SNS use was assessed by asking participants: "Please select your most frequently used media service at home (excluding study time, such as homework)." The response options included calling, messaging/chatting (e.g., LINE, KakaoTalk), watching TV, playing games, watching videos (e.g., YouTube), using apps (e.g., Instagram, X, Snapchat, Facebook), searching for information, watching cartoons, reading fiction, and others. Participants were then divided into two groups: SNS users (LINE, KakaoTalk, Instagram, X, Snapchat, and Facebook) and non-SNS users.

2.3.3. Screentime

Daily recreational screen-based activities, defined as media use for non-study purposes, was measured based on the Japanese Ministry's annual lifestyle habits survey for elementary school children (Ministry of Education, Culture, Sports, Science and Technology, 2024b). Participants were asked the question, "How many hours per day do you usually spend using TV, smartphones, tablets, game consoles, etc. at home? (excluding study time such as homework)." Answers were collected separately for weekdays and weekends using the following categories: "less than 1 h," "1–2 h," "2–3 h," and "more than 3 h." Average daily screentime was calculated using the following: (average weekday screen time × 5) + (average weekend screen time × 2)/7.

2.3.4. Body Size Perception and Preference

Body image was assessed by silhouette charts (Collins, 1991) to maintain children's engagement and facilitate responses. The charts contained seven silhouettes, ranging from very thin (a value of 1) to very obese (a value of 7). The Collins figures with facial features were performed by presenting the figures in order from 1 to 7. Participants were asked to select the silhouette that best represented their current body image (CBI) and IBI. The difference between CBI and IBI was calculated as the body size perception and preference (CBI − IBI). A body size perception and preference score ≥ 1 indicated that participants' "desired to be thinner"; a score < 1 indicated participants' "desired to be heavier"; and a score of 0 indicated that participants were satisfied with their bodies. Body size perception and preference has been validated for elementary school boys and girls (Troncone et al., 2018; Cuesta-Zamora & Navas, 2017).

2.3.5. Body Size Misperception

To assess body size misperception, participants categorized their body shape on a five-point scale: thin, slightly thin, normal, slightly overweight, or overweight. Body size misperception was calculated by comparing perceived body shape with actual body shape (Yumen et al., 2023). A body size misperception score < 1 was indicated underestimation, meaning a child with a normal body shape perceived themselves as thin/slightly thin or an overweight child perceived themselves as thin/slightly thin/or normal. A distortion score ≥ 1 was indicated overestimation, meaning an underweight child perceived themselves as normal/slightly overweight/ overweight, and normal body shape perceived as slightly overweight/overweight. A distortion score of 0 indicated no distortion, meaning that perceived body shape matched actual body shape. Body size misperception was previously validated in young adult populations (Yumen et al., 2023). In the present study, internal consistency was adequate (Cronbach's $\alpha = 0.93$ girls, 0.91 boys).

2.3.6. Ideal Body Image

Participants identified their IBI reference group based on relational closeness and included nobody, family members, close friends (i.e., those they regularly interact with), classmates (i.e., those they do not regularly interact with), and media figures (e.g., celebrities, models, idols, athletes, influencers, others on SNS). These classifications are those followed by Scully et al. (2023). Participants were asked to identify their ideal body image reference from the following options: "Nobody," "Family," "Close friends," "Classmates," or "Media figures." To transform this into an analyzable variable, we first set "Nobody" as the reference category (coded as 0). Each of the other responses ("Family," "Close friends," "Classmates," and "Media figures.") was recoded into a separate binary variable, with 1 indicating selection of that category and 0 otherwise. This approach allowed us to include these variables as a dependent variable in the logistic regression analyses. Internal consistency in this study was high (Cronbach's $\alpha = 0.97$ girls, 0.96 boys).

2.4. Data Analysis

Sex was dummy-coded (boy = 0, girl = 1), and missing data were removed using the listwise option. Group comparisons were conducted using Student's *t*-test, the Mann–Whitney U, or Chi-squared tests, as appropriate. Shapiro–Wilk tests confirmed that all variables except weight, height, and POW were non-normally distributed (all p's < 0.001). Therefore, Mann–Whitney U tests were used to compare sex differences and SNS users vs. non-SNS users. As most items exhibited group sex-based differences, all analyses accounted for sex. Hierarchical multivariate linear regression analyses were used to examine whether SNS use was uniquely associated with body size perception and preference and body size misperception. Multinomial logistic regression was conducted to assess the relationship between SNS use and IBI. The dependent variables included body size perception and preference, body size misperception, and IBI (criterion: nobody). The independent variable was SNS use (criterion: do not use). Because screen time, grade, and POW were considered as potentially confounding variables in the multivariate analysis (Kvardova et al., 2025), Model 1 used screen time, Model 2 used grade, and POW was added to Model 1 as an adjusting variable. The standardized coefficient (β) was calculated for hierarchical multivariate linear regression analyses. Conversely, the odds ratio was determined for multinomial logistic regression. Both analyses used 95% confidence intervals (95% CIs).

In hierarchical multivariate linear regression, assumption testing indicated non-normally distributed residuals in each model. Consequently, results were interpreted using nonparametric bootstrapping. No multicollinearity issues were detected (as all tolerance values were >0.87). For multinomial logistic regression, the Hosmer–Lemeshow was utilized to assess the model's goodness-of-fit. A priori power calculations were not conducted. However, a post hoc power analysis indicated sufficient power to detect significant associations when three covariates were included (hierarchical multivariate linear regression analyses: boy and girl, 0.99; multinomial logistic regression analyses: boy and girl, 0.99). The power of the unadjusted model was 0.83 for boys and 0.98 for girls.

All statistical analyses were conducted using the Statistical Package for the Social Sciences (SPSS) version 29 (IBM Inc., Tokyo, Japan). The significance level was set to $\alpha = 0.05$.

3. Results

3.1. Participant's Characteristics

The study included 611 boys and 650 girls. Compared to boys, girls more frequently used SNSs, especially LINE and KakaoTalk. Girls also reported a greater body size perception and preference and a stronger IBI. Conversely, boys had longer screen time and a greater body size misperception than girls (Table 1).

Table 1. Participants characteristics.

Physical Characteristics	Boy (n = 611)		Girl (n = 650)		p
Grade 3	n = 137		n = 164		
Height (cm) [1]		128.45 (5.28)		127.58 (5.97)	0.080
Weight (kg) [1]		26.96 (4.48)		26.72 (4.20)	0.958
POW [1,4]		−0.89 (11.97)		0.77 (11.17)	0.098
Grade 4	n = 179		n = 161		
Height (cm) [1]		132.7 (6.73)		133.20 (7.18)	0.959
Weight (kg) [1]		30.19 (5.82)		29.09 (5.02)	0.059
POW [1,4]		0.77 (16.80)		−1.64 (14.81)	0.156
Grade 5	n = 162		n = 155		
Height (cm) [1]		140.17 (6.83)		140.33 (7.92)	0.919
Weight (kg) [1]		35.80 (7.51)		33.94 (7.25)	**0.018**
POW [1,4]		2.45 (14.90)		−0.63 (14.14)	0.055
Grade 6	n = 133		n = 170		
Height (cm) [1]		146.37 (8.36)		147.95 (6.03)	**0.009**
Weight (kg) [1]		40.44 (10.38)		39.79 (6.37)	0.391
POW [1,4]		2.94 (20.01)		0.24 (13.91)	0.392
SNSs	Boy (n = 611)		Girl (n = 650)		p
Used SNSs [3]					**<0.001**
Yes		181 (29.6)		279 (42.9)	
No		430 (70.4)		371 (57.1)	
Contents [3]					
LINE, Kakao Talk					**<0.001**
Yes		165 (27.0)		265 (40.8)	
No		446 (73.0)		385 (59.2)	
Instagram, Snapchat					0.233
Yes		3.9 (24)		5.4 (35)	
No		96.1 (587)		94.6 (615)	
X, Facebook					1.000
Yes		3.1 (19)		3.2 (21)	
No		96.9 (592)		96.8 (629)	
Screentime (minutes) [2]		98.31 (64.29,132.86)		88.02 (47.14,115.71)	**<0.001**
Body Image	Boy (n = 611)		Girl (n = 650)		p
CBI [2,5]		3.89 (3.00,4.00)		3.83 (3.00,4.00)	0.100
IBI [2,5]		3.77 (3.00,4.00)		3.45 (3.00,4.00)	**<0.001**
Body size perception and preference [2,6]		0.12 (0.00,1.00)		0.38 (0.00,1.00)	**<0.001**
Body size misperception [2,7]		−0.31 (−1.00,0.00)		−0.18 (−1.00,0.00)	**0.007**
Ideal body image [3]					**<0.001**
Nobody		426 (69.7)		393 (60.5)	
Family		19 (3.1)		28 (4.3)	
Close friends		38 (6.2)		69 (10.6)	
Classmates		8 (1.3)		28 (4.3)	
Media figures		120 (19.6)		132 (20.3)	

Note. Abbreviations: POW, percentage of overweight; SNSs, social networking services; CBI, current body image; IBI, ideal body image. [1] Values represent mean (SD). p-values were analyzed via Student's t-test. [2] Values represent mean (IQR). p-values were analyzed via the Mann–Whitney U test. [3] Values represent n (%). p-values were analyzed by the Chi-square test. [4] POW (calculated from the standard weight by sex, age, and height used in the School Health Statistics Survey). [5] The score range is 1–7 (1 = very thin, 7 = very obese). [6] Body size perception and preference represents the difference between CBI and IBI (CBI−IBI). [7] The score range is −4–4 (<1 = underestimation, 0 = no distortion, >1 = overestimation). Bold: significant differences in p-Value.

3.2. Characteristics of SNS Users and Nonusers

SNS users were compared to nonusers regarding grade, obesity index, screen time, and body image constructs by sex. There were no group differences in both sexes' CBI, IBI, and body size perception and preference. Conversely, compared to the nonuser group, SNS users increased in grade level and had longer screen time. Body size misperception was less in SNS users than nonusers in girls. SNS users recorded less nobody values in IBI and more media figures than the nonuser group. This significant difference was not present in boys (Table 2).

Table 2. Characteristics of social networking service users and nonusers.

Item	Boy (n = 611)			Girl (n = 650)		
	SNS Users	Non-SNS Users	p	SNS Users	Non-SNS Users	p
Grade [3]						
3	16(8.8)	125(29.1)	**<0.001**	43(15.4)	122(32.9)	**<0.001**
4	45(24.9)	131(30.5)		55(19.7)	102(27.5)	
5	56(30.9)	102(23.7)		78(28.0)	81(21.8)	
6	64(35.4)	72(16.7)		103(36.9)	66(17.8)	
POW [1,4]	2.70(14.78)	0.55(17.24)	0.146	−0.08(12.80)	−0.71(13.21)	0.543
Screentime (minutes) [2]	106.95(72.86,153.21)	94.73(64.29,115.71)	**0.002**	106.95(47.14,115.71)	94.73(47.14,115.71)	**0.025**
CBI [2,5]	3.99(3.00,5.00)	3.85(3.00,4.00)	0.090	3.83(3.00,4.00)	3.82(3.00,4.00)	0.805
IBI [2,5]	3.78(3.00,4.00)	3.77(3.00,4.00)	0.900	3.78(3.00,4.00)	3.77(3.00,4.00)	0.961
Body size perception and preference [2,6]	0.22(0.00,1.00)	0.08(−1.00,1.00)	0.159	0.22(0.00,1.00)	0.08(0.00,1.00)	0.927
Body size misperception [2,7]	−0.33(−1.00,0.00)	−0.36(−1.00,0.00)	0.138	−0.20(0.00,0.00)	−0.36(−1.00,0.00)	**0.014**
Ideal body image [3]						
Nobody	114(63)	312(72.6)	0.109	150(53.8)	243(65.5)	**0.004**
Family	5(2.8)	14(3.3)		14(5)	14(3.8)	
Close friends	16(8.8)	22(5.1)		36(12.9)	33(8.9)	
Classmates	2(1.1)	6(1.4)		8(2.9)	20(5.4)	
Media figures	44(24.3)	76(17.7)		71(25.4)	61(16.4)	

Note. Abbreviations: POW, percentage of overweight; SNSs, social networking services; CBI, current body image; IBI, ideal body image. [1] Values represent mean (SD). p-values were analyzed via Student's t-test.[2] Values represent mean (IQR). p-values were analyzed via the Mann–Whitney U test. [3] Values represent n (%). p-values were analyzed by the Chi-square test. [4] POW (calculated from the standard weight by sex, age, and height used in the School Health Statistics Survey). [5] The score range is 1–7 (1 =very thin, 7 =very obese). [6] Body size perception and preference represents the difference between CBI and IBI (CBI−IBI). [7] The score range is −4–4 (<1 = underestimation, 0 = no distortion, >1= overestimation). Bold: significant differences in p-value.

3.3. Associations of Body Image with SNS Use

After adjustments for grade, obesity index, and screen time, it was found that SNS use was not significantly associated with body size perception and preference or body size misperception in boys. Because of the IBI, SNS use was associated with close friends and media of IBI when adjusting for screen time. Furthermore, SNS use was not associated with close friends after adjusting for grade, obesity index, and screen time. Conversely, media figures remained a significant predictor of SNS use.

After adjustments for grade, obesity index, and screen time, SNS use was found not to be associated with body size perception and preference in girls. However, when including screen time, SNS use did not significantly correlate with body size misperception, but this relationship disappeared after adjusting for grade and POW. The IBI result showed that SNS use was associated with close friends and media figures when including screen time. Furthermore, similar to boys, SNS use by girls was not associated with close friends after adjusting for grade and POW, while media figures remained a statistically significant predictor of SNS use (Table 3).

Table 3. Associations of body image with social networking services use.

Outcomes Dependent Variables	Univariate Analysis		Multivariate Analysis (Model 1)		Multivariate Analysis (Model 2)	
	β/OR [95%CI]	SE	β/OR [95%CI]	SE	β/OR [95%CI]	SE
Boys (n = 611)						
Body size perception and preference [1]	0.06 [−0.04, 0.29]	0.09	0.05 [−0.06, 0.29]	0.09	0.03 [−0.09, 0.22]	0.08
Body size misperception [1]	0.07 [−0.01, 0.30]	0.08	0.07 [−0.01, 0.30]	0.08	0.04 [−0.09, 0.24]	0.08
Ideal body image [2]						
Nobody	1		1		1	
Family	0.98 [0.34, 2.78]	0.53	0.98 [0.34, 2.81]	0.54	1.08 [0.36, 3.20]	0.55
Close friends	2.00 [1.01, 3.92] *	0.35	1.92 [0.97, 3.81]	0.35	1.74 [0.86, 3.55]	0.36
Classmates	0.91 [0.18, 4.59]	0.82	1.10 [0.22, 5.58]	0.83	1.52 [0.27, 8.44]	0.87
Media figures	1.58 [1.03, 2.43] *	0.22	1.71 [1.11, 2.65] *	0.22	1.64 [1.04, 2.57] *	0.23
Girls (n = 650)						
Body size perception and preference [1]	0.01 [−0.13, 0.16]	0.07	0.00 [−0.14, 0.15]	0.07	−0.01 [−0.15, 0.13]	0.07
Body size misperception [1]	0.09 [0.02, 0.28] *	0.07	0.08 [0.00, 0.26] *	0.07	0.04 [−0.07, 0.20]	0.07
Ideal body image [2]						
Nobody	1		1		1	
Family	1.62 [0.75, 3.49]	0.39	1.60 [0.74, 3.47]	0.39	1.93 [0.87, 4.30]	0.41
Close friends	1.77 [1.06, 2.96] *	0.26	1.74 [1.04, 2.92] *	0.26	1.56 [0.91, 2.67]	0.27
Classmates	0.65 [0.28, 1.51]	0.43	0.64 [0.28, 1.50]	0.43	0.61 [0.25, 1.45]	0.45
Media figures	1.89 [1.27, 2.81] **	0.20	1.87 [1.25, 2.78] *	0.20	1.72 [1.14, 2.60] *	0.21

Note. N = 1261. * $p < 0.05$, ** $p < 0.01$. Abbreviations: SNSs, social networking services; β, standardized coefficient; OR, odds ratio; CIs, confidence intervals; SE, standard error. β/OR, the results of the β calculation using continuous variables (body size perception and preference and body size misperception) and the OR calculation using binary dependent variables (ideal body image). [1] Values represent β [95% CI]. p-values were analyzed via linear regression analysis. β values are standardized beta values from the non-bootstrapped model; SE and CI are from the bootstrapped model. [2] Values represent OR [95% CI]. p-values were analyzed via multinomial logistic regression analysis. Model 1: Effect estimates adjusted for screen time. Model 2: Model 1 + grade and POW. Ideal body image criterion: Nobody.

4. Discussion

While studies continue to accumulate suggesting that SNS use poses a risk to children's body image, the majority of these studies have been conducted with late adolescents and young adults. This study examined the relationship between SNS use and body image in preadolescents.

The findings indicate that SNS use does not directly contribute to body size perception and preference in Japanese preadolescents. These findings contradict prior results from an Australian sample of girls aged 10–12, wherein girls who reported using SNSs reported higher body surveillance, greater body size perception and preference, more dieting behaviors, and a greater thin-ideal internalization compared to nonusers (Tiggemann & Slater, 2014). Similarly, a study on preadolescent US girls reported that appearance-focused SNS use exacerbated negative body image concerns (Markey & Daniels, 2022). Furthermore, prior studies on adolescents have identified moderate correlations between SNS use and body satisfaction (Jarman et al., 2021; Karam et al., 2023). SNSs serve as a primary source of appearance-related pressure, influencing body esteem through thin-ideal internalization and body comparison, both of which worsen body size perception and preference in adolescents (Roberts et al., 2022). Moreover, adolescents encounter various developmental challenges during early to middle adolescence (Rodgers & Rousseau, 2022). Adolescence is a critical period for social comparison and body image sensitivity, and many studies reported that physical comparisons are made with friends and upward social interaction. This results in heightened body size perception and preference.

Body image concerns and body size perception and preference are independent of time spent on SNSs, browsing friends' SNSs profiles, viewing users' photos and statuses, and liking and commenting among male and female American college students (Kim & Chock, 2015), and Instagram among young females (Pedalino & Camerini, 2022), which are related to the purpose of SNSs and the activities performed on them. However, the absence of a significant association in this study suggests that the purpose of SNS use and the content they are exposed to may not shape body ideals as strongly in preadolescents compared to in adolescents and that they may respond differently to appearance activities on social media concerning their body size perception and preference. For example, children may prefer platforms wherein physical comparisons are less likely to be made with the child's favorite animal, character, food, or game-related content. Regardless, preadolescents need to establish a correct body image for themselves before puberty to reduce body size perception and preference, which is likely to occur with age. Regardless, most studies on SNS use and body image have predominantly focused on girls, adolescents, and young adults. Limited studies have examined the effects of SNS use on boys or the potential effects of different SNS platforms or cultural variations. While this study included boys in childhood, further investigation remains necessary to understand this issue.

We found that SNS use was significantly associated with body size misperception in girls but not in boys. Girls who used SNSs exhibited higher levels of body size misperception than nonusers. A study focusing on body size misperception among adolescents showed that both moderate and high levels of smartphone dependency were linked to body size misperception (Cho et al., 2024). Moreover, SNS use affecting body size misperception has been found in preadolescent girls (Daniels & Robnett, 2021). Our findings align with previous research targeting preadolescents or adolescents (Hosseini & Padhy, 2023; Cho et al., 2024; Kwon et al., 2022; Jung & Jun, 2022), suggesting that frequent exposure to diverse body images on SNSs disrupts conventional standards and intensifies self-evaluation distortions. However, this result was neither found in boys nor did it persist in girls after adjusting for grade and the obesity index. This suggests that the influence of SNSs on body image is complex and varies by sex, age, and body type. Mental health-related factors such as depression and anxiety are also known to be significantly associated with body size misperception in 13–17-year-olds (Derenne & Beresin, 2018). This effect may intensify as adolescence approaches. However, studies on SNS use and body size misperception remain limited, and the mechanisms involved have not been clarified. A more detailed examination of SNS usage patterns, including frequency and content, is needed to clarify these effects.

This study found who the IBI belongs to in preadolescence, which revealed that SNS use strongly correlated with admiration for media figures in both sexes. This suggests that media influence outweighs other social influences (e.g., family, friends, classmates). Although traditional media studies have known that media including television and magazines shape the IBI both preadolescents and adolescents (Piran et al., 1999; Keery et al., 2004; Lovering et al., 2018; Rodgers et al., 2011), the spread of SNSs may amplify this effect. Unlike those of celebrities and models in traditional media, images on SNSs may appear to be realistic comparisons for adolescent girls (Choukas-Bradley et al., 2022). Furthermore, interestingly, appearance comparisons with others of the same-gender peers rather than with models reinforce the internalization of ideal image standards in female adolescents (Moriyasu et al., 2012). Basically, body comparisons with others and with friends may reinforce the desire to lose weight and increase dieting behavior. These findings highlight that even in childhood media portrayals exert a broader influence on body image than direct peer interactions. Notably, these media-driven ideals perpetuate unrealistic standards and could be one of the factors driving SNS use as children attempt to conform their appearance to these ideals.

This consistent association across sexes underscores the universal impact of media, although the IBI may differ between boys and girls. Both preadolescent and adolescent boys typically aspire to a muscular body shape (Pope et al., 2000a; Tylka, 2011; Ricciardelli & Yager, 2015), whereas preadolescent and adolescent girl idealize a thin, beautiful body shape (Hargreaves & Tiggemann, 2004; Oehlhof et al., 2009), or an appearance that is both thin and muscular in adolescence (Roberts et al., 2022). These sex differences emerge even in childhood, and future research on SNSs and body image should include sex-specific measures of body size misperception, including differences in SNS use content, satisfaction with musculature, and IBI.

While this study contributes to the limited body of research on SNS use and body image in preadolescents, several limitations warrant mention. First, the cross-sectional design precludes causal interpretations as establishing temporal relationships is difficult. Future longitudinal studies are necessary to determine whether SNS use predicts body image concerns among children. The findings may also not generalize to other countries and cultures, which have different body ideals and risks to preadolescents' health behaviors. It will be interesting to examine the effect of cultural differences on preadolescents' body image in further research.

As a limitation in measurement, the classification of SNS use was binary, and differences based on the detailed content types of SNSs could not be examined. The present study indicates that 36.5% of children used SNSs; however, their SNS use likely varied. Some preadolescents used SNSs for visual content (e.g., Instagram and TikTok), for viewing other people's photos, and for communication, such as for messaging their friends. Thus, the type of SNSs content that directly associates with children's body image is not clear. Additionally, photo-based SNSs content likely includes both appearance-focused (e.g., selfies) and non-appearance-focused (e.g., pets) posts. Some preadolescents used SNSs for appearance purposes, such as visually oriented social media like Instagram, TikTok, and Snapchat, for viewing other people's photos, and for communication, such as for messaging their friends. Thus, the type of SNSs content that directly associates with children's body image is not clear. Future research should examine and differentiate between the photo-based and non-photo-based SNSs content that children share to better understand this issue among preadolescents. Moreover, children's engagement level was not assessed in the present study. Investigating children's psychological and social dimensions could provide valuable insights for enhancing educational settings and refining instructional approaches. Therefore, these variables should be included as measurement items in future research.

Despite these limitations, this study provides important insights that will help guide specific groups of children in using SNSs appropriately and reducing body size perception and preference, body size misperception, and excessive weight loss.

5. Conclusions

This study could not confirm an association between SNS use and body size perception and preference among children. However, whilst our findings suggest that SNS use was not linked to body size perception and preference, it may contribute to body size misperception in girls. Additionally, for both boys and girls, SNS use was strongly associated with greater body image admiration for media figures than for their immediate friends and classmates. The present study contributes to the understanding of SNS use and body size perception and preference, body size misperception, and IBI in preadolescent boys and girls, offering insights for future work on this crucial aspect of preadolescent body image.

SNS use can negatively impact body size perception and preference in preadolescents, but there is a lack of research enlightening the particular mechanisms that underlie this relationship. Efforts to reduce SNS use even before adolescence will be critical in supporting the development of a healthy body image in future adolescents. Consistently, gaining insight into how SNS use contributes to body image is key for advancing research in this area and informing prevention efforts aimed at reducing body size perception and preference in preadolescents. In Japan, research on the effects of SNSs on body image for children remains in its early stages. We hope that future research will determine the extent to which engaging with body image content on SNSs can affect body image in children.

Author Contributions: Conceptualization, A.B. and N.O.; Methodology, A.B.; Validation, A.B., M.S., R.Y. and Y.I.; Formal Analysis, A.B.; Investigation, A.B., M.S., R.Y. and Y.I.; Data Curation, A.B. and N.O.; Writing—Original Draft Preparation, A.B.; Writing—Review and Editing, A.B., M.S., R.Y., Y.I. and N.O.; Supervision, N.O.; Project Administration, N.O.; Funding Acquisition, N.O. All authors have read and agreed to the published version of the manuscript.

Funding: This research received no external funding. The APC was funded by the University of Tsukuba.

Institutional Review Board Statement: The study was conducted in accordance with the Declaration of Helsinki, and the protocol was approved by the Ethics Committee of the Faculty of Health and Sports Sciences at the University of Tsukuba (No: 023-144) on 19 April 2024.

Informed Consent Statement: Informed consent was obtained from all individual participants included in the study. Written informed consent was obtained from the parents.

Data Availability Statement: Restrictions apply to the availability of these data due to the inclusion of sensitive or confidential information such as the height and weight of prepubescent children. Data were obtained from Gakuen no Mori Compulsory Education School and are available from the authors with the permission of Gakuen no Mori Compulsory Education School.

Acknowledgments: We would like to thank the children, their parents, and their teachers in the survey.

Conflicts of Interest: The authors declare no conflicts of interest.

References

British Medical Association. (2000). *Eating disorder, body image & the media* (D. R. Morgan, Ed.). BMJ Publishing Group.

Bucchianeri, M. M., Arikian, A. J., Hannan, P. J., Eisenberg, M. E., & Neumark-Sztainer, D. (2013). Body dissatisfaction from adolescence to young adulthood: Findings from a 10-year longitudinal study. *Body Image, 10*(1), 1–7. [CrossRef] [PubMed]

Cho, H., Park, J., Lee, D., & Shin, D. W. (2024). Association of body image distortion with smartphone dependency and usage time in adolescents: A cross-sectional Korean youth study. *Korean Journal of Family Medicine. advance online publication.* [CrossRef]

Choukas-Bradley, S., Roberts, S. R., Maheux, A. J., & Nesi, J. (2022). The perfect storm: A developmental–sociocultural framework for the role of social media in adolescent girls' body image concerns and mental health. *Clinical Child and Family Psychology Review, 25*(4), 681–701. [CrossRef]

Collins, M. E. (1991). Body figure perceptions and preferences among preadolescent children. *International Journal of Eating Disorders, 10*(2), 199–208. [CrossRef]

Common Sense. (2022). *The Common Sense Census: Media use by tweens and teens, 2021.* Available online: https://www.commonsensemedia.org/sites/default/files/research/report/8-18-census-integrated-report-final-web_0.pdf (accessed on 3 July 2025).

Cuesta-Zamora, C., & Navas, L. (2017). A review of instruments for assessing body image in preschoolers. *Universal Journal of Educational Research, 5*(10), 1667–1677. [CrossRef]

Dane, A., & Bhatia, K. (2023). The social media diet: A scoping review to investigate the association between social media, body image and eating disorders amongst young people. *PLoS Glob Public Health, 3*(3), e0001091. [CrossRef]

Daniels, E. A., & Robnett, R. (2021). The STEM pipeline: Do media and self-objectification create an early exit for middle school girls? *The Journal of Early Adolescence*, *41*(7), 1099–1124. [CrossRef]

Derenne, J., & Beresin, E. (2018). Body image, media, and eating disorders—A 10-year update. *Academic Psychiatry*, *42*, 129–134. [CrossRef] [PubMed]

Dixon, R., Adair, V., & O'Connor, S. (1996). Parental influences on the dieting beliefs and behaviors of adolescent females in New Zealand. *Journal of Adolescent Health*, *19*(4), 303–307. [CrossRef] [PubMed]

Duggan, M., & Smith, A. (2013). *Social media update 2013*. Pew research internet project. Available online: http://www.pewinternet.org/2013/12/30/social-media-update-2013/ (accessed on 3 July 2025).

Fukuoka City Official Website. (2025a). *City profile*. Available online: https://www.city.fukuoka.lg.jp/shisei/profile/index.html/ (accessed on 25 April 2025). (In Japanese).

Fukuoka City Official Website. (2025b). *Fukuoka city estimated population*. Available online: https://www.city.fukuoka.lg.jp/soki/tokeichosa/shisei/toukei/jinkou/jinnkousokuhou.html/ (accessed on 25 April 2025). (In Japanese).

Grogan, S. (2016). *Body image: Understanding body dissatisfaction in men, women and children* (3rd ed.). Routledge. [CrossRef]

Hansson, E., & Schmidt, M. (2025). Measuring disordered eating in adolescent boys: A systematic literature review. *Eating Disorders. Online ahead of print*. [CrossRef]

Hargreaves, D. A., & Tiggemann, M. (2004). Idealized media images and adolescent body image: "Comparing" boys and girls. *Body Image*, *1*(4), 351–361. [CrossRef]

Holland, G., & Tiggemann, M. (2016). A systematic review of the impact of the use of social networking sites on body image and disordered eating outcomes. *Body Image*, *17*, 100–110. [CrossRef] [PubMed]

Hosseini, S. A., & Padhy, R. K. (2023). Body image distortion (archived). In *StatPearls*. StatPearls Publishing.

Huang, Q., Peng, W., & Ahn, S. (2021). When media become the mirror: A meta-analysis on media and body image. *Media Psychology*, *24*(4), 437–489. [CrossRef]

Ibaraki Prefectural Government. (2022). *2020 population census basic population results report*. Available online: https://www.pref.ibaraki.jp/kikaku/tokei/fukyu/tokei/betsu/jinko/kokucho/kokucho2020/documents/kokucho2020-report.pdf (accessed on 3 July 2025). (In Japanese).

Japan Society of School Health. (2015). *Health checkup manual for students*. Available online: https://www.gakkohoken.jp/book/ebook/ebook_H270030/index_h5.html#1 (accessed on 3 July 2025). (In Japanese).

Japan Sports Agency. (2024). *Results of the 2024 nationwide survey on physical fitness, motor skills, and exercise habits*. Available online: https://www.mext.go.jp/sports/b_menu/toukei/kodomo/zencyo/1411922_00013.html/ (accessed on 25 April 2025). (In Japanese).

Jarman, H. K., Marques, M. D., McLean, S. A., Slater, A., & Paxton, S. J. (2021). Motivations for social media use: Associations with social media engagement and body satisfaction and well-being among adolescents. *Journal of Youth and Adolescence*, *50*(12), 2279–2293. [CrossRef] [PubMed]

Jung, E. H., & Jun, M. K. (2022). Factors affecting body image distortion in adolescents. *Children*, *9*(12), 1944. [CrossRef]

Karam, J. M., Bouteen, C., Mahmoud, Y., Tur, J. A., & Bouzas, C. (2023). The relationship between social media use and body image in Lebanese university students. *Nutrients*, *15*(18), 3961. [CrossRef] [PubMed]

Keery, H., Van Den Berg, P., & Thompson, J. K. (2004). An evaluation of the tripartite influence model of body dissatisfaction and eating disturbance with adolescent girls. *Body Image*, *1*(3), 237–251. [CrossRef]

Kim, J. W., & Chock, T. M. (2015). Body image 2.0: Associations between social grooming on Facebook and body image concerns. *Computers in Human Behavior*, *48*, 331–339. [CrossRef]

Kvardova, N., Machackova, H., Maes, C., & Vandenbosch, L. (2025). Navigating beauty standards on social media: Impact of appearance activity on adolescents' body dissatisfaction. *Journal of Youth and Adolescence. online ahead of print*. [CrossRef]

Kwon, S., Kim, R., Lee, J. T., Kim, J., Song, S., Kim, S., & Oh, H. (2022). Association of smartphone use with body image distortion and weight loss behaviors in Korean adolescents. *JAMA Network Open*, *5*(5), e2213237. [CrossRef]

Liechty, J. M. (2010). Body image distortion and three types of weight loss behaviors among nonoverweight girls in the United States. *Journal of Adolescent Health*, *47*(2), 176–182. [CrossRef]

Lovering, M. E., Rodgers, R. F., George, J. E., & Franko, D. L. (2018). Exploring the tripartite influence model of body dissatisfaction in postpartum women. *Body Image*, *24*, 44–54. [CrossRef]

Mabe, A. G., Forney, K. J., & Keel, P. K. (2014). Do you "like" my photo? Facebook use maintains eating disorder risk. *International Journal of Eating Disorders*, *47*(5), 516–523. [CrossRef] [PubMed]

Markey, C. H., & Daniels, E. A. (2022). An examination of preadolescent girls' social media use and body image: Type of engagement may matter most. *Body Image*, *42*, 145–149. [CrossRef]

Ministry of Education, Culture, Sports, Science and Technology. (2024a). *2024 school health statistics survey results*. Available online: https://www.e-stat.go.jp/stat-search/files?page=1&toukei=00400002&tstat=000001011648/ (accessed on 25 April 2025). (In Japanese)

Ministry of Education, Culture, Sports, Science and Technology. (2024b). *Overview of the 2024 national survey of academic achievement*. Available online: https://www.nier.go.jp/24chousakekkahoukoku/report/data/24summary.pdf (accessed on 3 July 2025). (In Japanese)

Ministry of Internal Affairs and Communications. (2021). *Information and communications in Japan*. Available online: https://www.soumu.go.jp/johotsusintokei/whitepaper/eng/WP2021/2021-index.html/ (accessed on 25 April 2025).

Miyazaki, Y., & Ogata, T. (2006). Psychological features and nutritional assessment of female university students with a tendency toward Eeating disorders. *The Japanese Journal of Nutrition and Dietetics*, *64*(1), 31–43. (In Japanese). [CrossRef]

Mobile Society Research Institute. (2023). *2023 Parents and children survey*. Available online: https://www.moba-ken.jp/project/children/kodomo20240606.html (accessed on 3 July 2025). (In Japanese).

Mohsenpour, M. A., Karamizadeh, M., Barati-Boldaji, R., Ferns, G. A., & Akbarzadeh, M. (2023). Structural equation modeling of direct and indirect associations of social media addiction with eating behavior in adolescents and young adults. *Scientific Reports*, *13*(1), 3044. [CrossRef] [PubMed]

Moriyasu, K., Moroi, K., Maehara, S., & Kogirima, M. (2012). Drive for thinness and social comparison (1): Moderating effects of thin-ideal internalization. *DWCLA Human Life and Science*, *45*, 29–36. (In Japanese) [CrossRef]

Murata, M., & Ito, K. (2003). Report of research on nutrition, exercise and recreation from the viewpoint of health and QOL in children, supported by Health, Labour and Welfare for research on Health Services in 2002. In M. Murata (Ed.), *On the optimal weight in school-age children* (pp. 10–13). Doshisha Women's College of Liberal Arts. (In Japanese) [CrossRef]

Nagata, J. M., Brown, T. A., Murray, S. B., & Lavender, J. M. (Eds.). (2021). *Eating disorders in boys and men*. Springer International Publishing. [CrossRef]

Neumark-Sztainer, D., Wall, M. M., Chen, C., Larson, N. I., Christoph, M. J., & Sherwood, N. E. (2018). Eating, activity, and weight-related problems from adolescence to adulthood. *American Journal of Preventive Medicine*, *55*(2), 133–141. [CrossRef]

Oehlhof, M. E., Musher-Eizenman, D. R., Neufeld, J. M., & Hauser, J. C. (2009). Self-objectification and ideal body shape for men and women. *Body Image*, *6*(4), 308–310. [CrossRef]

Patton, G. C., & Viner, R. (2007). Pubertal transitions in health. *The Lancet*, *369*(9567), 1130–1139. [CrossRef]

Pedalino, F., & Camerini, A. L. (2022). Instagram use and body dissatisfaction: The mediating role of upward social comparison with peers and influencers among young females. *International Journal of Environmental Research and Public Health*, *19*(3), 1543. [CrossRef]

Piran, N., Levine, M., & Steiner-Adair, C. (Eds.). (1999). *Preventing eating disorders: A handbook of interventions and special challenges* (1st ed.). Routledge. [CrossRef]

Pope, H. G., Gruber, A. J., Mangweth, B., Bureau, B., Decol, C., Jouvent, R., & Hudson, J. I. (2000a). Body image perception among men in three countries. *American Journal of Psychiatry*, *157*(8), 1297–1301. [CrossRef]

Pope, H. G., Pope, H., Phillips, K. A., & Olivardia, R. (2000b). *The adonis complex: The secret crisis of male body obsession*. Simon and Schuster. [CrossRef]

Rapee, R. M., Oar, E. L., Johnco, C. J., Forbes, M. K., Fardouly, J., Magson, N. R., & Richardson, C. E. (2019). Adolescent development and risk for the onset of social-emotional disorders: A review and conceptual model. *Behaviour Research and Therapy*, *123*, 103501. [CrossRef]

Ricciardelli, L. A., & McCabe, M. P. (2002). Psychometric evaluation of the body change inventory: An assessment instrument for adolescent boys and girls. *Eating Behaviors*, *3*(1), 45–59. [CrossRef]

Ricciardelli, L. A., & Yager, Z. (2015). *Adolescence and body image: From development to preventing dissatisfaction*. Routledge.

Roberts, S. R., Maheux, A. J., Hunt, R. A., Ladd, B. A., & Choukas-Bradley, S. (2022). Incorporating social media and muscular ideal internalization into the tripartite influence model of body image: Towards a modern understanding of adolescent girls' body dissatisfaction. *Body Image*, *41*, 239–247. [CrossRef]

Rodgers, R. F., Chabrol, H., & Paxton, S. J. (2011). An exploration of the tripartite influence model of body Dissatisfaction and disordered eating among Australian and French college women. *Body Image*, *8*(3), 208–215. [CrossRef]

Rodgers, R. F., & Rousseau, A. (2022). Social media and body image: Modulating effects of social identities and user characteristics. *Body Image*, *41*, 284–291. [CrossRef]

Rodgers, R. F., Slater, A., Gordon, C. S., McLean, S. A., Jarman, H. K., & Paxton, S. J. (2020). A biopsychosocial model of social media use and body image concerns, disordered eating, and muscle-building behaviors among adolescent girls and boys. *Journal of Youth and Adolescence*, *49*, 399–409. [CrossRef]

Saiphoo, A. N., & Vahedi, Z. (2019). A meta-analytic review of the relationship between social media use and body image disturbance. *Computers in Human Behavior, 101*, 259–275. [CrossRef]

Sato, Y., & Tsuchiya, S. (2010). Eating disorder tendency in high school students: Gender differences. *Japanese Journal of Psychosomatic Medicine, 50*(4), 321–326. (In Japanese) [CrossRef]

Scully, M., Swords, L., & Nixon, E. (2023). Social comparisons on social media: Online appearance-related activity and body dissatisfaction in adolescent girls. *Irish Journal of Psychological Medicine, 40*(1), 31–42. [CrossRef]

Sharma, A., & Vidal, C. (2023). A scoping literature review of the associations between highly visual social media use and eating disorders and disordered eating: A changing landscape. *Journal of Eating Disorders, 11*(1), 170. [CrossRef]

Shulman, S. (1993). Close relationships and coping behavior in adolescence. *Journal of Adolescence, 16*(3), 267–283. [CrossRef]

Smahel, D., Machackova, H., Mascheroni, G., Dedkova, L., Staksrud, E., Ólafsson, K., Livingstone, S., & Hasebrink, U. (2020). *EU Kids Online 2020: Survey results from 19 countries*. EU Kids Online. [CrossRef]

Smith, A. R., Hames, J. L., & Joiner, T. E., Jr. (2013). Status update: Maladaptive Facebook usage predicts increases in body dissatisfaction and bulimic symptoms. *Journal of Affective Disorders, 149*(1–3), 235–240. [CrossRef]

Tiggemann, M., & Slater, A. (2014). NetTweens: The internet and body image concerns in preteenage girls. *The Journal of Early Adolescence, 34*(5), 606–620. [CrossRef]

Troncone, A., Cascella, C., Chianese, A., Galiero, I., Zanfardino, A., Confetto, S., Perrone, L., & Iafusco, D. (2018). Changes in body image and onset of disordered eating behaviors in youth with type 1 diabetes over a five-year longitudinal follow-up. *Journal of Psychosomatic Research, 109*, 44–50. [CrossRef]

Tsukuba City Official Website. (2025). *Tsukuba City overview*. Available online: https://www.city.tsukuba.lg.jp/shisei/joho/index.html/ (accessed on 26 April 2025). (In Japanese).

Tylka, T. L. (2011). Renement of the tripartite influence model for men: Dual body image pathways to body change behaviors. *Body Image, 8*(3), 199–207. [CrossRef]

Vandenbosch, L., & Eggermont, S. (2016). The interrelated roles of mass media and social media in adolescents' development of an objectified self-concept: A longitudinal study. *Communication Research, 43*(8), 1116–1140. [CrossRef]

Vannatta, K., Gartstein, M. A., Zeller, M., & Noll, R. B. (2009). Peer acceptance and social behavior during childhood and adolescence: How important are appearance, athleticism, and academic competence? *International Journal of Behavioral Development, 33*, 303–311. [CrossRef]

Webb, H. J., & Zimmer-Gembeck, M. J. (2014). The role of friends and peers in adolescent body dissatisfaction: A review and critique of 15 years of research. *Journal of Research on Adolescence, 24*(4), 564–590. [CrossRef]

Yumen, Y., Takayama, Y., Hanzawa, F., Sakane, N., & Nagai, N. (2023). Association of social networking sites use with actual and ideal body shapes, and eating behaviors in healthy young Japanese women. *Nutrients, 15*(7), 1589. [CrossRef]

Zhang, J., Wang, Y., Li, Q., & Wu, C. (2021). The relationship between SNS usage and disordered eating behaviors: A meta-analysis. *Frontiers in Psychology, 12*, 641919. [CrossRef]

European Journal of
Investigation in Health, Psychology and Education

MDPI

Article

Exploring Traditional and Cyberbullying Profiles in Omani Adolescents: Differences in Internalizing/Externalizing Symptoms, Prosocial Behaviors, and Academic Performance

Ahmed Al Saidi [1,2], Claudio Longobardi [3,*], Matteo Angelo Fabris [3], Sofia Mastrokoukou [4] and Shanyan Lin [3]

1 Department of Behavioral Sciences Methodology, University of Valencia, 46010 Valencia, Spain; a.alsaidi@squ.edu.om
2 Department of Child Health, Sultan Qaboos University, P.O. Box 50, Al-Khoudh P.C. 123, Oman
3 Department of Psychology, University of Turin, 10123 Turin, Italy; matteoangelo.fabris@unito.it (M.A.F.); shanyan.lin@unito.it (S.L.)
4 Department of Political and Social Scineces, University of Salerno, 84084 Fisciano, Italy; smastrokoukou@unisa.it
* Correspondence: claudio.longobardi@unito.it

Abstract: In the digital age, adolescents spend considerable time online, heightening their exposure to both cyberbullying and traditional bullying. However, few studies have investigated both forms of victimization simultaneously, particularly regarding their impact on adolescents in Middle Eastern countries such as Oman. This study used latent profile analysis to identify victimization profiles based on indicators of verbal, social, physical, and cyberbullying victimization. The participants included 1204 Omani students (604 girls, 50.2%; M = 14.04, SD = 0.20, aged 14–15). Three victimization profiles emerged: (1) non-victims (n = 989, 82.1%), (2) traditional victims (n = 156, 13.0%), and (3) dual victims (n = 59, 4.9%). The BCH approach revealed that adolescents in the non-victims profile, with the lowest levels of both traditional and cyberbullying victimization, reported the lowest levels of internalizing (M = 10.14, SD = 0.11) and externalizing symptoms (M = 10.36, SD = 0.10) and the highest academic performance (M = 4.59, SD = 0.02), whereas their prosocial behaviors were relatively low (M = 4.71, SD = 0.08). Adolescents in the traditional victims' profile had moderate levels on nearly all outcomes. Adolescents in the dual victims' profile, who experienced both traditional and cyberbullying, reported the highest levels of behavioral symptoms ($M_{internalizing}$ = 11.94, $SD_{internalizing}$ = 0.34; $M_{externalizing}$ = 12.81, $SD_{externalizing}$ = 0.38) and prosocial behaviors (M = 5.63, SD = 0.36), along with the lowest academic performance (M = 4.37, SD = 0.11). These findings underscore the need for culturally sensitive, multi-level interventions to protect Omani adolescents from both traditional and cyberbullying and to support their academic and psychosocial well-being.

Keywords: bullying victimization; cyberbullying; Omani adolescent; internalizing symptoms; externalizing symptoms; prosocial behaviors; academic performance

1. Introduction

School is an important context for the cognitive, emotional, and relational development of adolescents (Fabris et al., 2023). However, different forms of violence can occur in this context, especially among peers (Longobardi et al., 2017, 2019a, 2021). Among the forms of peer victimization in the school context, one of the most widespread and that attracts particular attention in the educational and academic field is certainly bullying, which still represents a social emergency today (Fabris et al., 2021; Longobardi et al., 2019b; Thornton et al., 2024). We use the term bullying to refer to the intentional and repeated harming of a person where there is an actual or perceived power imbalance between the victim(s) and the perpetrator(s) (Hellström et al., 2021). By traditional bullying (TB), we mean a form of victimization that takes place in a real-life context, often face-to-face, and includes forms of physical victimization (hitting, kicking, pushing and shoving), verbal victimization (name-calling, teasing, and threats) or social victimization (spreading rumors and social isolation).

However, with the advent of new technologies, and, in particular, the proliferation of smartphones and easy access to the internet for adolescents, a new form of bullying has emerged in the online environment, known as cyberbullying (CB) (Fabris et al., 2022; Morese et al., 2024). Although TB and CB are conceptually similar and share different characteristics, the two forms of bullying also have distinctive features (H. J. Thomas et al., 2015). Traditional bullying typically occurs during school hours and in specific physical contexts. In contrast, cyberbullying transcends these boundaries, exposing victims to potential harm 24 h a day, 7 days a week. Furthermore, in traditional bullying, the victim knows the identity of their aggressors, whereas in cyberbullying, the identity of the attackers may be unknown to the victim, and the number of people witnessing the forms of victimization can be exponentially higher than in TB. Estimating the prevalence of (cyber)bullying victimization is not straightforward, as estimates can vary not only due to contextual and cultural differences, but especially due to different measurement strategies (Moore et al., 2017). Indeed, it is estimated that between 10 and 35 percent of adolescents have experienced traditional bullying (Li et al., 2024), while about 15 percent have experienced forms of victimization through cyberbullying (Jadambaa et al., 2019; Modecki et al., 2014). Furthermore, a recent meta-analysis (Li et al., 2024) estimated that one-third of adolescent victims of traditional bullying also tend to experience online victimization, while as many as two-thirds of CB victims also experience TB. This reflects the fact that TB is a strong predictor of CB and that a large percentage of cyber-victims are also victimized in an offline context. This is not surprising given that, at least in adolescence, the dynamics and quality of relationships experienced with peers in the offline environment appear to mirror and shape relationships in the online environment. Indeed, in the online world, adolescents might mainly keep in touch and interact with people from the real world, as in the case of class WhatsApp groups (Lin et al., 2025; Marengo et al., 2021). Therefore, it is possible that those who have poor relationships with peers in the physical/offline environment and are bullied by peers also do so in the online environment. However, data on the prevalence of bullying victimization and cyberbullying victimization are predominantly focused on Western cultures, especially Europe and the United States, while research has only recently focused on under-researched geographic areas, such as the Middle East.

In order to better understand how these forms of victimization are interrelated and influenced by broader factors, recent theoretical and cross-cultural studies offer valuable insights. Recent contributions to the literature have emphasized the importance of viewing traditional and cyberbullying as interconnected processes rather than as independent phenomena. Keith et al. (2025) proposed a socio-developmental trajectory in which adolescents involved in traditional bullying increasingly transfer aggressive behaviors to digital spaces, especially as peer interactions move online and group norms shift. This transition is facilitated by mechanisms such as digital disinhibition, anonymity, and the amplification of peer visibility through social media platforms. Similarly, C. Wang et al. (2024), through a longitudinal investigation, demonstrated that students who engage in offline aggression during middle school are more likely to become cyber aggressors or cyber victims by the end of high school, suggesting a fluid and reciprocal pathway between offline and online peer dynamics. These models point to dual victimization not as a simple accumulation of risks, but as a complex and evolving experience shaped by adolescents' broader social ecology and digital literacy.

Moreover, cross-cultural studies have increasingly revealed that the prevalence, perception, and impact of bullying vary across regions because of differences in sociocultural norms, parental mediation, and digital access. Saleem et al. (2025), in a comparative study between Middle Eastern and South Asian adolescents, found that collectivist values, gender norms, and family involvement played a critical role in moderating the likelihood and psychological impact of cyberbullying victimization. Gallego-Jiménez and Rodríguez Otero (2025) further showed that school-based peer aggression in Southern European contexts differs in form and reporting patterns when compared with Northern European samples, particularly regarding cyberbullying. These findings highlight the need for localized research on dual victimization, particularly in under-studied areas like Oman, where cultural, religious, and technological frameworks may uniquely shape the experience of peer victimization. Incorporating such perspectives allows for a more ecologically valid and culturally sensitive interpretation of bullying dynamics and strengthens the theoretical contributions of this study within the global literature.

Beyond prevalence and definitions, an essential area of concern involves how victimization affects adolescents' psychological and academic outcomes. There is a large body of research that shows how bullying and cyberbullying can affect students' school adjustment and emotional well-being. By school adjustment, we mean a range of outcomes that affect not only academic performance (GPA), but also emotional–behavioral well-being at school (internalizing and externalizing symptoms) and better relationships with others (prosocial behavior). Several longitudinal and cross-sectional studies have documented the association between traditional bullying (Samara et al., 2021) and cyberbullying (Gardella et al., 2017; Wright, 2015) and poor academic performance in adolescence. It is possible that adolescents who are bullied tend to lose self-confidence and have low aspirations, and that depressive feelings can reduce concentration and energy to devote to learning. In addition, victimization can increase feelings of isolation and cause the young person to perceive the school environment as dangerous and frustrating, leading to high levels of absenteeism and truancy. It is clear that this situation is not optimal for the student's academic journey and would significantly limit their learning opportunities. Although the literature suggests that both bullying and cyberbullying victimization are associated with poorer academic performance in adolescents, some data suggest that those who suffer from both forms of victimization perform worse than those who suffer from only one of the forms of victimization (Rostam-Abadi et al., 2024).

Another element that could characterize the school adjustment is prosocial behavior. By prosocial behavior, we mean social behavior that benefits other people or society as a whole and manifests itself in behaviors such as helping, sharing, donating, cooperating, and volunteering (Eisenberg et al., 2006). Prosocial behaviors are important in the school context because they allow children and adolescents to more easily build and establish positive relationships with peers, fostering greater integration into the class group (Longobardi et al., 2021), which, in turn, is a protective factor for victimization (Fu et al., 2023; Z. Wang et al., 2024). In this direction, Fu et al. (2023) found that low levels of prosocial behaviors in children and adolescents were directly and indirectly associated with the risk of TB, while no significant association was found with CB. However, other studies have indicated that adolescent victims of CB tend to act in a less prosocial way when they witness CB episodes as bystanders (Cao & Lin, 2015) and tend to become perpetrators themselves (Völlink et al., 2013). For example, it is possible that previous victimization experiences may lead to an increase in mistrust of others, as well as feelings of revenge and negative emotions among those affected, which could discourage prosocial behaviors in favor of more antisocial behaviors. Some data suggest that victims of CB are more likely to seek help from peers, parents, or teachers when they exhibit higher levels of prosocial behaviors (Holfeld & Mishna, 2019). Nevertheless, we must keep in mind that victims of CB tend to be isolated and have poor social skills (Marengo et al., 2024), which limits opportunities to develop higher levels of prosocial behaviors (Lin et al., 2024). However, not all studies agree. For example, Geng et al. (2022) found that adolescents who exhibit more altruistic behaviors online are also those who are more at risk of CB, whereas Kaiser et al. (2020) reported that although adolescents who were victims of cyberbullying exhibited higher prosocial behaviors than cyberbullies, they did so at a comparable level to their peers who were not involved in cyberbullying. In addition, several lines of evidence suggest that adolescents who are victims of bullying (Kokkinos & Kipritsi, 2012) or cyberbullying (Fabris et al., 2023) tend to show high levels of empathy compared to aggressors or uninvolved peers, which is an important precursor to prosocial behavior. These findings might appear counterintuitive, particularly given the elevated psychological distress observed in dual victims. One possible explanation is that, in collectivist contexts such as Oman, adolescents may adopt prosocial behaviors as a coping mechanism to restore social harmony or gain peer acceptance. This aligns with findings in other collectivist societies, such as Jordan (Shahrour et al., 2020), Saudi Arabia (AlBuhairan et al., 2017), and South Korea (Lee et al., 2022), where social cohesion and conformity are emphasized. Alternatively, the result could be influenced by social desirability biases typical in self-report measures, as suggested in studies from Iran and Pakistan (Saleem et al., 2025). These competing explanations call for further investigation using mixed-methods designs to clarify whether such prosocial tendencies reflect authentic behaviors, adaptive strategies, or reporting artifacts. These data seem to suggest that previous experiences of victimization may make adolescents more sensitive and attentive to the emotional needs and pleas for help of those in a situation of distress or danger. Thus, the link between prosocial behavior and victimization is important, but more research is needed to understand the nature and direction of this association.

Finally, bullying and cyberbullying are generally associated with an increase in psychological distress, which is associated with an increase in internalized symptoms (such as anxiety, depression, and suicidal ideation) and externalized symptoms (such as hyperactivity, conduct disorder, and substance use) (Prino et al., 2019). Research suggests that TB is associated with increased internalizing (Gini et al., 2018) or externalizing symptoms (Eastman et al., 2018; Marengo et al., 2018), while some evidence suggests that bullying victims report both symptoms (Eastman et al., 2018; Lin et al., 2024; Prino et al., 2019). However, a recent meta-analysis (Casper & Card, 2017) found that forms of peer victimization (both overt and relational) tended to be more strongly associated with internalizing symptoms than externalizing symptoms. This may be due to the fact that peer victimization during adolescence creates a greater sense of isolation from the group at a developmental stage when a sense of belonging to the group is crucial to adolescents' emotional well-being, which also reduces internalizing symptoms, such as suicidal ideation (Longobardi et al., 2020). Peer victimization could thus lead the individual to reflect on their social failures, leading them to social withdrawal, a greater sense of loneliness, and fear of future victimization, thus undermining the possibility of building meaningful relationships with peers and developing appropriate social skills. Furthermore, a recent study found that internalizing symptoms are more associated with being a victim of bullying, whereas internalizing symptoms seem to better characterize the so-called bully-victims (Valente et al., 2024). Regarding victimization by CB, the literature shows similar results. Indeed, several studies show an association between CB victimization and an increase in internalizing symptoms (Elgar et al., 2014; Marengo et al., 2024) and externalizing symptoms (Fisher et al., 2016). In particular, a meta-analysis of longitudinal studies (Marciano et al., 2020) showed that not only does cyberbullying victimization predict both symptom areas, but that only internalizing symptoms predict the risk of becoming a victim of cyberbullying longitudinally. However, a more recent 3-year longitudinal study (Holfeld & Mishna, 2019) found, after controlling for TB victimization, that CB victimization was associated with both internalizing and externalizing symptoms and that both symptomatology (internalizing and externalizing) predicted CB victimization, not vice versa.

Although several studies have demonstrated an association between CB and TB victimization and measures of psychological well-being, few studies have focused on dual victimization, i.e., simultaneous victimization in offline and online contexts. These data seem to indicate that adolescents who are victimized in both contexts tend to have greater psychological distress than those who were only victimized in offline or only online (Ossa et al., 2023; Pengpid & Peltzer, 2023) and, in particular, report higher levels of internalizing symptoms (Chudal et al., 2021; Holfeld & Mishna, 2019; Pengpid & Peltzer, 2023; Schneider et al., 2012) and a greater tendency towards deviant behavior (K. J. Thomas & McCuddy, 2020) and risky behavior (Ossa et al., 2023; Pengpid & Peltzer, 2023; Rostam-Abadi et al., 2024).

Aims of This Study

Although the Middle East region has been identified as a particularly vulnerable region for bullying in schools (Ran et al., 2023), much research is still needed to understand the prevalence of TB and CB in this geographical area and its potential impact on adolescents' school performance and psychological adjustment. In particular, our study focuses on adolescent students in Oman, as this country is one of the Middle Eastern countries most affected by bullying in schools, according to the limited data available to us. In fact, according to the World Health Organization's Global School-based Students Health Survey (GSHS) (see Abdalmaleki et al., 2022), bullying affects 47 percent of Omani students, while it affects 22.8 percent of students in the United Arab Emirates and 28 percent in Kuwait. Therefore, the aim of this cross-sectional study is to use latent profile analysis to identify victimization profiles based on indicators of verbal, social, physical, and cyberbullying victimization. In addition, we test whether there are differences in school adjustment (academic performance, prosocial behavior, and internalizing and externalizing symptoms) based on the identified clusters.

2. Materials and Methods

2.1. Participants and Procedure

The participants included 1204 students (grades 9 and 10) recruited from public schools in the capital of Oman (Muscat). There were 604 girls (50.2%) in this convenience sample. The average age of the sample was 14.04 (SD = 0.20), ranging from 14 to 15 years old. More detailed demographic information is provided in Table 1. There are no specific sample size guidelines for latent profile analysis (LPA), and a sample size between 300 and 1000 is generally considered sufficient for the commonly used fit-in indices to work adequately (Nylund-Gibson & Choi, 2018). The sample size in the current study slightly exceeded this range, which may have facilitated the identification of profiles with relatively low prevalence. The research plan was approved by the authors' affiliated university (n. 0592463). This study strictly adhered to the ethical principles outlined in the Declaration of Helsinki, with all participants treated in accordance with ethical guidelines for research involving human subjects. Before data collection, the participants and their parents or legal guardians had to sign a consent form. The participants were assured of the confidentiality of the data and were informed that participation in this study was voluntary. They could refuse to participate in this study at any time or withdraw from this study if they felt uncomfortable answering any question.

Table 1. Participants' characteristics of demography.

		Frequency	Percentage
Father education	Cannot read and write	26	2.2%
	Primary school	138	11.5%
	Secondary school	916	76.1%
	College	78	6.5%
	Postgraduate	46	3.8%
Mother education	Cannot read and write	8	0.7%
	Primary school	40	3.3%
	Secondary school	1044	86.7%
	College	111	9.2%
	Postgraduate	1	0.1%
Monthly income [A]	325–500	44	3.7%
	501–900	313	26.0%
	901–1200	606	50.3%
	1201 and above	241	20.0%
Parent status	Live together	1199	99.6%
	Divorced	5	0.4%

Note: [A] The currency unit here is Omani Rials.

2.2. *Measures*

2.2.1. Adolescent Peer Relations Instrument (APRI; Parada, 2000)

Traditional bullying victimization was measured by the victimization part of the APRI (Parada, 2000). There are 18 items in this part that measure three dimensions of traditional bullying victimization, including verbal victimization (6 items, e.g., "I was teased by students saying things to me"), social victimization (6 items, e.g., "A student wouldn't be friends with me because other people didn't like me"), and physical victimization (6 items, e.g., "Students crashed into me on purpose as they walked by"). The students were required to rate all the items on a six-point Likert response scale (1 = Never, 6 = Every day). The sum of all the ratings was calculated and taken as the final score for traditional victimization, with a higher value indicating more victimization. The Cronbach's alphas of the APRI were 0.80 (verbal victimization), 0.83(social victimization), and 0.76 (physical victimization).

2.2.2. Revised Cyber Bullying Inventory-II (RCBI-II; Topcu & Erdur-Baker, 2018)

Cyberbullying victimization was measured by the RCBI-II (Topcu & Erdur-Baker, 2018). There are 10 items in the victimization section (beginning phrase "It happened to me" and "On the Internet") of the RCBI-II (e.g., "sending embarrassing or hurtful messages"). The students were asked to rate these 10 items on a 4-point scale (1 = Never, 2 = Once, 3 = Twice or three times, 4 = More than three times). The final score for cyberbullying was calculated as the sum of all the ratings, which ranged from 10 to 40. The confirmatory factor analysis revealed an acceptable structural validity of the RCBI-II in this study: $\chi^2/df = 4.81$, RMSEA = 0.06, CFI = 0.99, TLI = 0.97, SRMR = 0.03. The Cronbach's alpha of the RCBI-II victimization section was 0.84.

2.2.3. The Strengths and Difficulties Questionnaire (SDQ; R. Goodman, 1997)

The self-reported version of the SDQ (R. Goodman, 1997) was used to measure the students' internalizing symptoms, externalizing symptoms, and prosocial behaviors. In the SDQ, there are 25 items in 5 subscales, including emotional symptoms (5 items, e.g., "I am often unhappy, depressed or tearful"), peer relationship problems (5 items, e.g., "I am usually on my own"), behavioral problems (5 items, e.g., "I am often accused of lying or cheating"), hyperactivity (5 items, e.g., "I am easily distracted"), and prosocial behaviors (5 items, e.g., "I am helpful if someone is hurt, upset or feeling ill"). The students were asked to rate their behavioral symptoms and prosocial behaviors on a 3-point scale (0 = Not true, 1 = Somewhat true, and 2 = Certainly true). In line with the approach recommended by A. Goodman et al. (2010), the internalizing symptoms score (ranging from 0 to 20) was calculated by summing the peer relationship problems and emotional symptoms subscale scores. Similarly, the externalizing symptoms score (also ranging from 0 to 20) was calculated by combining the scores from the behavioral problems and hyperactivity subscales. The Cronbach's alphas were 0.71 (internalizing symptoms), 0.70 (externalizing symptoms), and 0.76 (prosocial behaviors).

2.2.4. Academic Performance

The teachers were asked to provide an assessment of each student's overall academic performance by reporting their average grade across all school subjects. Each subject was evaluated using a standardized 5-point grading scale, where scores ranged from 1 to 5: 1 represented "Not Accepted", 2 represented "Accepted", 3 indicated "Good", 4 represented "Very Good", and 5 signified "Excellent". Higher scores on this scale corresponded to higher levels of academic achievement, resulting in a cumulative average grade that reflected each student's overall GPA.

2.3. Data Analysis

Data analysis was conducted using SPSS 29 and Mplus 8.3. To identify the profiles of traditional and cyberbullying victimization among Omani adolescents, we employed LPA with verbal victimization, social victimization, physical victimization, and cybervictimization as indicators. Models with varying profile numbers, from one to five, were analyzed to determine the optimal profile structure. Several criteria were used to evaluate model fit, including (1) Akaike information criterion (AIC), (2) Bayesian information criterion (BIC), (3) adjusted Bayesian information criterion (aBIC), (4) entropy ($\geq$0.7, Reinecke, 2006), (5) the Lo–Mendell–Rubin adjusted likelihood ratio test, (6) the bootstrapped likelihood ratio test (BLRT), and (7) minimum profile size ($\geq$5% of the total sample, Marsh et al., 2009). Substantive interpretability, utility, and classification diagnostics were also considered in selecting the final model (Nylund-Gibson & Choi, 2018). To compare behavioral symptoms and academic performance means across the latent profiles, we applied the BCH approach (Asparouhov & Muthén, 2014). This method was selected as optimal for evaluating mean differences between profiles, allowing for an overall chi-square test followed by multiple pairwise comparisons.

3. Results

3.1. The Identified Victimization Profiles

To identify traditional and cyberbullying victimization profiles among Omani adolescents, latent profile analysis was conducted. Profile numbers ranging from 1 to 5 were tested, and the results are presented in Table 2. As shown in the table, the model with three profiles fits the data relatively well compared to the other models. Specifically, its LMR was significant, indicating that the three-profile model provided a better fit than the two-profile model. Its entropy was above 0.7, and the sample size in the smallest profile was above 50 and close to 5%. In addition, in the four-profile model, the LMR was nonsignificant, suggesting it did not improve upon the five-profile model. Therefore, the model with three profiles was selected as the final model.

Table 2. Fit indices for bullying victimization profiles.

Number of Profiles	AIC	BIC	aBIC	Entropy	LMR	BLRT	Smallest Profile
One Profile	28,873.906	28,914.653	28,889.242	–	–	–	100% (n = 1204)
Two Profiles	26,341.997	26,408.212	26,366.918	0.989	2472.204 ***	2541.909 ***	0.15532 (n = 187)
Three Profiles	25,401.787	25,493.468	25,436.293	0.979	924.154 **	950.210 ***	0.04900 (n = 59)
Four Profiles	25,041.278	25,158.427	25,085.370	0.983	950.210	370.509 ***	0.01246 (n = 15)
Five Profiles	24,692.513	24,835.128	24,746.189	0.982	348.928	358.766 ***	0.01163 (n = 14)

Note: AIC = Akaike information criterion, BIC = Bayesian information criterion, aBIC = adjusted BIC, LMR = Lo–Mendell–Rubin adjusted likelihood ratio test, BLRT = bootstrapped likelihood ratio test; ** $p < 0.01$, *** $p < 0.001$.

The z-scores of the indicators in each profile are illustrated in Figure 1 to better depict the characteristics of each group. As shown, Profile 1 (n = 989, 82.1%) represents the largest group, comprising students with all victimization z-scores below the average level. This profile was labeled as "non-victims". Profile 2 (n = 156, 13.0%) was the second-largest group, where all indicators were positive, and the level of cybervictimization in this profile was relatively lower than the three forms of traditional victimization. This profile was labeled as "traditional victims". Profile 3 (n = 59, 4.9%), as the smallest group, included students with the highest levels across all victimization types, including verbal, social, physical, and cybervictimization, relative to the other profiles, earning the label "dual victims".

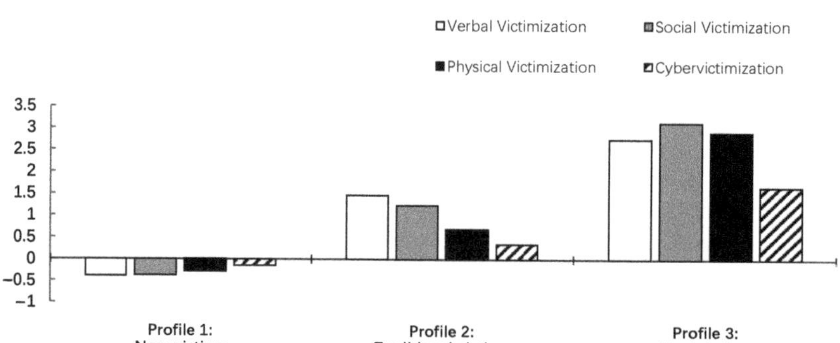

Figure 1. Z-scores of the indicators in each profile. Note, the longitudinal axis is the z-score of each indicator.

3.2. The Victimization Profiles and Profile Differences

To examine profile differences in internalizing and externalizing symptoms, prosocial behaviors, and academic performance, the BCH approach (Asparouhov & Muthén, 2014) was employed. The results are presented in Table 3. Significant differences were found between the profiles across all studied variables: internalizing symptoms (Wald's χ^2 = 25.32, df = 2, $p < 0.001$), externalizing symptoms (Wald's χ^2 = 44.16, df = 2, $p < 0.001$), prosocial behaviors (Wald's χ^2 = 7.68, df = 2, $p < 0.05$), and GPA (Wald's χ^2 = 14.19, df = 2, $p < 0.01$). Pairwise comparisons showed that the students in the non-victims profile (Profile 1) had the lowest levels of internalizing and externalizing symptoms, the lowest prosocial behaviors, and the highest GPA. The students in the traditional victims profile (Profile 2) exhibited moderate internalizing symptoms and had levels of externalizing symptoms and prosocial behaviors similar to Profile 1, with GPA similar to Profile 3 and relatively low. The dual victims profile (Profile 3) displayed the highest levels of internalizing and externalizing symptoms, the lowest academic performance, and the highest level of prosocial behaviors.

Table 3. Mean differences in the studied variables between bullying victimization profiles.

	M (SD)			Mean Difference	
Outcomes	Profile 1: Non-Victims (n = 989)	Profile 2: Traditional Victims (n = 156)	Profile 3: Dual Victims (n = 59)	Overall Test Wald's χ^2 (df = 2)	Pairwise Comparison
SDQ_Internalizing symptoms	10.14 (0.11)	10.76 (0.26)	11.94 (0.34)	25.32 ***	P3 > P2 > P1
SDQ_Externalizing symptoms	10.36 (0.10)	9.94 (0.20)	12.81 (0.38)	44.16 ***	P3 > P2, P3 > P1, P2 ≈ P1
SDQ_Prosocial behaviors	4.71 (0.08)	4.94 (0.17)	5.63 (0.36)	7.68 *	P3 > P1, P1 ≈ P2, P2 ≈ P3
GPA	4.59 (0.02)	4.31 (0.08)	4.37 (0.11)	14.19 **	P1 > P2, P1 > P3, P2 ≈ P3

Note. P1 = Profile 1, P2 = Profile 2, P3 = Profile 3; * $p < 0.05$, ** $p < 0.01$, *** $p < 0.001$.

4. Discussion

Bullying and cyberbullying as forms of peer victimization are still a current social emergency. However, research on the prevalence and associated risk factors has mainly focused on Western countries, particularly Americans and Europeans, while only recently has interest in this topic begun to grow in previously under-researched geographical areas such as Middle Eastern countries, including Oman, in particular. Our study attempts to move in this direction and identify traditional and cyberbullying victimization profiles among Omani youth. We are not aware of any other similar studies in Oman.

From the analyses, three distinct profiles emerged that characterize the sample of adolescents examined, referred to as "non-victims" (profile 1), "traditional victims" (profile 2), and "dual victims" (profile 3). "Non-victims" represents the broadest profile and comprises around 82 percent of young people. This profile is characterized by adolescents who have experienced no or minimal victimization in any type of bullying or cyberbullying victimization. This finding seems to indicate that a large percentage of Omani adolescents are not exposed to any experience of bullying or cyberbullying, which is more positive than in other cultural contexts and seems to contradict the limited data available, according to which about half of Omani adolescents report at least one experience of peer victimization (Abdalmaleki et al., 2022). However, we must bear in mind that research on the prevalence of bullying in the cultural context of the Middle East is still underdeveloped, and cultural and methodological factors may play a role. For example, some scholars (Ginanjar et al., 2024) have pointed out that Arabic terms referring to bullying can have positive connotations and therefore do not always define bullying as a negative act. In Oman, the term bullying is known as "Suluk Audwani", which describes a person who attacks another with their tongue or a weapon. Although this term evokes aggression towards another person, it seems to refer almost exclusively to a physical attack and underestimates the existence of forms of social and verbal bullying, which could have an impact on the prevalence of bullying reported by children and adolescents. In addition, Arab cultures tend to emphasize values such as courage, honor, and protecting one's family and community, which may discourage adolescents from reporting bullying (Al Saadoon et al., 2024). The second largest group is the "traditional victims", who represent 13 percent of the sample. This group is so named because the adolescents in this group have been exposed to peer victimization and, in particular, report high scores on all three forms of TB victimization (physical, verbal, and social) but low scores on CB victimization. Thus, the adolescent students in this group are characterized by having experienced traditional forms of bullying, but do not tend to report experiences of cyberbullying victimization. Finally, the third profile is labeled "dual victims" and represents approximately 5 percent of the sample involved. Adolescents in this sample have been exposed to all types of victimization and have high levels, including cyberbullying. Thus, these youth show high levels of TB victimization (physical, verbal, and social) and CB victimization. These data appear to be consistent with emerging trends in the literature, which suggest that traditional bullying is still more prevalent than cyberbullying (Jadambaa et al., 2019; Modecki et al., 2014). However, they also reflect the finding that the majority of adolescents who are victims of cyberbullying are simultaneously bullied in the offline world, while only a quarter of adolescents who experience TB are also victims of cyberbullying (Li et al., 2024).

In addition, our data attempted to understand the differences between the profiles in terms of school adjustment by measuring differences in the dimensions of academic performance, emotional and behavioral well-being (internalizing and externalizing symptoms), and prosocial behavior. Adolescents in Profile 2 (traditional victims) tended to have moderate levels of internalizing disorders and, similar to the dual victims, lower levels of academic achievement compared to the adolescents who were not exposed to bullying (Profile 1—non-victims). These data can be understood on the basis of previous literature. In particular, there is evidence that bullying victimization tends to be more strongly associated with internalizing symptoms than with externalizing symptoms (Casper & Card, 2017; Valente et al., 2024). It is possible that the experience of bullying increases a sense of low hope, isolation, and low self-esteem and fears of future victimization in victimized adolescents and thus promotes the occurrence of internalizing symptoms (Prino et al., 2019). In addition, the feeling of loneliness and reduced contact with peers could lead to unmet needs for belonging and closeness to the group, which increases the risk of internalizing symptoms (Casper & Card, 2017; Longobardi et al., 2020). The link between bullying victimization and internalizing symptoms may be particularly strong in Omani adolescents, considering that Oman is considered a collectivist culture. Therefore, harmony and group affiliation are highly valued in this cultural context, and experiences of victimization may reinforce perceptions of isolation and loneliness, making the link between victimization and internalizing symptoms particularly salient in this cultural context. However, there is evidence that adolescents with internalizing symptoms have characteristics that make them more likely to be targeted by aggressors, such as a greater tendency to isolate, greater introversion and poor social skills, which also make them less able to respond to bullying and defend themselves effectively (Valente et al., 2024). In addition, the Profile 2 (traditional victims) and Profile 3 (dual victims) subjects show low levels of academic performance compared to the Profile 1 subjects. These data are consistent with the literature, indicating that stress related to the experience of victimization can impair attention and motivation, thereby decreasing the likelihood of academic success (Gardella et al., 2017; Samara et al., 2021). In addition, it is possible that adolescents who are victimized by peers tend to avoid school in order to avoid interacting with the perpetrators of violence directed at them, thereby reducing not only the opportunities to build relationships with peers in the class group but also the opportunity for learning.

Finally, our study shows that the adolescents in Profile 3 (dual victims) are those who exhibit higher levels of psychological distress (they reported higher levels of internalizing and externalizing symptoms) and higher levels of prosocial behavior. The fact that the latter group reported higher levels of externalizing symptoms than Profile 2 may indicate that CB victimization tends to be equally associated with internalizing and externalizing symptoms (Fisher et al., 2016; Marciano et al., 2020). In general, the fact that the adolescents in Profile 3 reported higher levels of psychological symptoms is consistent with the literature indicating that adolescents exposed to both forms of victimization (CB and TB), rather than just one of the two, have poorer mental health outcomes (Pengpid & Peltzer, 2023). It is possible that adolescents exposed to both forms of victimization have difficulty finding a safe place as they are simultaneously victimized in offline and online contexts. In this way, it is possible that these adolescents may experience increased distress and feelings of loneliness and reduced opportunities to develop a sense of group belonging and more functional emotion regulation strategies, leading to an increase in psychological distress. In addition, the data show that adolescents who experience both forms of victimization exhibit higher levels of prosocial behavior. This finding warrants further examination, and we must keep in mind that the literature on the relationship between prosocial behavior and peer victimization is articulate, and the data are not always consistent. However, there is evidence that adolescents who report altruistic behavior online are at higher risk of being victims of cyberbullying (Geng et al., 2022). Other research instead suggests that adolescents who have experienced forms of peer victimization (both in online and offline contexts) tend to report more empathy (Fabris et al., 2023; Kokkinos & Kipritsi, 2012), which is a precursor to prosocial behavior.

In this regard, recent findings suggest that the elevated prosocial behaviors observed in dual victims may be interpreted through the lens of empathy-based responses. Sobol et al. (2025) highlight that some bullied adolescents, particularly those who are also bystanders or dual victims, may display heightened sensitivity to others' suffering and adopt prosocial behaviors as a form of coping or self-protection. This behavioral pattern may serve to enhance social connectedness or reduce the risk of further victimization, especially in adolescents who feel vulnerable or isolated. Thus, the increased prosociality in dual victims may not simply reflect dispositional traits but rather a compensatory strategy shaped by their experiences of peer victimization. This behavior could also be encouraged by the particular cultural context in which belonging and group harmony, as well as prosocial behavior towards family and peers, are particularly valued. These authors hypothesize that previous victimization experiences have likely made victimized individuals more sensitive to the expression of others' suffering, resulting in increased prosocial behaviors. However, further studies are needed to understand these differences and the mechanisms involved. Furthermore, in our study, higher levels of prosocial behavior were found only in the dual victims' group, whereas the subjects in the traditional victims group showed similar levels to subjects in the non-victims group. Future studies should therefore investigate whether these differences are due to a more severe condition related to the presence of both forms of victimization (TB and CB) or whether the simultaneous presence of one form of victimization (especially online) determines these results.

5. Limitations of This Study and Future Research

Our study contributes to the understanding of the extent of the phenomenon of bullying/cyberbullying among adolescents in Oman, but our findings must be considered with the methodological limitations of this study in mind. As our study is cross-sectional, causal relationships between variables cannot be inferred from our analyses. For this reason, future replications in the context of longitudinal research projects are required. In addition, our research protocol included only quantitative self-report instruments. These instruments are valuable and widely used in this area of research, but they suffer from potential limitations in terms of social desirability, text comprehension, and the ability to correctly recall one's memories. Future studies could include different measures and other observers. In addition, future studies could enrich the protocol with qualitative questions to elicit more subjective reflections from participants. Finally, although the sample is numerically sufficient for the analysis, it cannot be considered representative of the population of Omani adolescents. Future studies could therefore invest in recruiting representative samples and include both early and late adolescents. Finally, we suggest comparing the data from this sample with subjects of other ages (e.g., young adults or primary school children) or making comparisons with adolescents from other cultural contexts or adolescents with special needs to understand the possible role of cultural and socio-demographic variables.

Practical Implications

Our study points to some possible practical implications, especially for teachers, educators, and psychologists dealing with adolescents. First, the fact that a significant percentage of adolescents have experienced forms of bullying and/or cyberbullying suggests the need to continue working in educational and school contexts, both at the level of prevention and intervention, in order to create more respectful and inclusive contexts and protect young victims. In addition, for young people with poor school adjustment, it is important to consider the possibility that forms of peer victimization are associated with it. On the other hand, for those who have been exposed to bullying and cyberbullying, it is important to consider how such experiences might be related to poor school adjustment and to intervene in the most vulnerable areas, such as psychological well-being, school performance, or interpersonal relationships. These findings suggest the importance of implementing differentiated intervention strategies tailored to the specific needs of the identified victim profiles. In particular, adolescents classified as dual victims—who report high levels of both traditional and cyber victimization along with increased psychological distress and elevated prosocial behavior—represent a high-risk group requiring targeted and multi-level interventions. For this subgroup, it is essential to design integrated programs that address emotional regulation, social skills training, and cognitive–behavioral support, with the goal of reducing internalizing/externalizing symptoms while promoting adaptive coping strategies. Furthermore, this study's results highlight the need to extend intervention frameworks beyond the school setting to include the family context. Recent research (Amin et al., 2024; Chu & Chen, 2024) has demonstrated the protective role of family-based factors—such as parental monitoring of online activity, open communication about peer relationships, and parental modeling of emotional competence—in reducing the risk of both traditional and cyber victimization. Embedding parent-focused components in school-based programs could enhance the efficacy of interventions by fostering consistent messages and support structures across home and school environments. For instance, structured parental workshops on digital literacy and emotion-focused parenting may serve as critical levers in mitigating adolescent vulnerability to peer victimization. Finally, our data could provide information for the training and awareness-raising of professionals working with young people in different capacities. This implies the necessity for intersectoral collaboration among schools, families, and, potentially, digital platform stakeholders to co-construct evidence-based, systemic prevention models. Such collaborative approaches are increasingly supported in the literature as effective means of addressing the multifactorial nature of bullying and cyberbullying phenomena, especially in socio-cultural contexts where digital behaviors and parenting practices may differ.

6. Conclusions

Despite the aforementioned limitations, our study contributes to the current literature by providing insight into the extent of bullying and cyberbullying victimization among adolescents in Oman. In particular, our study shows that a proportion of adolescents are exposed to both forms of traditional bullying and cyberbullying (dual victims) and that this group of adolescents has poorer school adjustment than those who are only exposed to traditional bullying.

Author Contributions: Conceptualization, C.L.; methodology, S.L.; software, S.L.; validation, S.L., S.M. and C.L.; formal analysis, S.L.; investigation, A.A.S.; resources, A.A.S.; data curation, A.A.S.; writing—original draft preparation, S.L., M.A.F. and A.A.S.; writing—review and editing, C.L. and S.M.; visualization, M.A.F.; supervision, C.L.; project administration, C.L. and A.A.S. All authors have read and agreed to the published version of the manuscript.

Funding: This research received no external funding.

Institutional Review Board Statement: This study was conducted in accordance with the Declaration of Helsinki and approved by the Ethics Committee of Università degli studi di Torino (protocol code 0592463 and date of approval: 2 November 2023).

Informed Consent Statement: Informed consent was obtained from all subjects involved in this study.

Data Availability Statement: The data that support the findings of this study are available from the corresponding author upon reasonable request.

Conflicts of Interest: The authors declare that they have no known competing financial interests or personal relationships that could have appeared to influence the work reported in this study.

Abbreviations

The following abbreviations are used in this manuscript:

TB	Traditional Bullying
CB	Cyberbullying
LPA	Latent Profile Analysis
GSHS	Global School-based Students Health Survey
APRI	Adolescent Peer Relations Instrument
RCBI-II	Revised Cyberbullying Inventory-II
SDQ	Strengths and Difficulties Questionnaire
GPA	Grade Point Average
SPSS	Statistical Package for the Social Sciences
AIC	Akaike Information Criterion
BIC	Bayesian Information Criterion
aBIC	Adjusted Bayesian Information Criterion
LMR	Lo–Mendell–Rubin Adjusted Likelihood Ratio Test

References

Abdalmaleki, E., Abdi, Z., Isfahani, S. R., Safarpoor, S., Haghdoost, B., Sazgarnejad, S., & Ahmadnezhad, E. (2022). Global school-based student health survey: Country profiles and survey results in the eastern Mediterranean region countries. *BMC Public Health, 22*(1), 130. [CrossRef] [PubMed]

AlBuhairan, F., Abou Abbas, O., El Sayed, D., Badri, M., Alshahri, S., & De Vries, N. (2017). The relationship of bullying and physical violence to mental health and academic performance: A cross-sectional study among adolescents in Kingdom of Saudi Arabia. *International Journal of Pediatrics and Adolescent Medicine, 4*(2), 61–65. [CrossRef] [PubMed]

Al Saadoon, M., Eltayib, R. A. A., Alhaj, A. H., Chan, M. F., Aldhafri, S., & Al-Adawi, S. (2024). The perception and roles of school mental health professionals regarding school bullying (Suluk Audwani) in Oman: A qualitative study in an urban setting. *International Journal of Environmental Research and Public Health, 21*(8), 991. [CrossRef] [PubMed]

Amin, A. N., Supartini, Y., Tambunan, E. S., Sulastri, T., Ningsih, R., & Hapsari, D. C. (2024). Analysis of factors that influence bullying behavior in adolescents in public middle school in East Jakarta Region. *Jurnal Keperawatan, 9*(2), 282–293. [CrossRef]

Asparouhov, T., & Muthén, B. (2014). Auxiliary variables in mixture modeling: Using the BCH method in Mplus to estimate a distal outcome model and an arbitrary secondary model. *Mplus Web Notes, 21*(2), 1–22.

Cao, B., & Lin, W. Y. (2015). How do victims react to cyberbullying on social networking sites? The influence of previous cyberbullying victimization experiences. *Computers in Human Behavior, 52*, 458–465. [CrossRef]

Casper, D. M., & Card, N. A. (2017). Overt and relational victimization: A meta-analytic review of their overlap and associations with social–psychological adjustment. *Child Development, 88*(2), 466–483. [CrossRef]

Chu, X., & Chen, Z. (2024). The associations between parenting and bullying among children and adolescents: A systematic review and meta-analysis. *Journal of Youth and Adolescence, 54*(4), 928–954. [CrossRef]

Chudal, R., Tiiri, E., Brunstein Klomek, A., Ong, S. H., Fossum, S., Kaneko, H., Kolaitis, G., Lesinskiene, S., Li, L., Huong, M. N., Praharaj, S. K., Sillanmäki, L., Slobodskaya, H. R., Srabstein, J. C., Wiguna, T., Zamani, Z., Sourander, A., & Eurasian Child Mental Health Study (EACMHS) Group. (2021). Victimization by traditional bullying and cyberbullying and the combination of these among adolescents in 13 European and Asian countries. *European Child & Adolescent Psychiatry, 31*, 1391–1404. [CrossRef]

Eastman, M., Foshee, V., Ennett, S., Sotres-Alvarez, D., Reyes, H. L. M., Faris, R., & North, K. (2018). Profiles of internalizing and externalizing symptoms associated with bullying victimization. *Journal of Adolescence, 65*, 101–110. [CrossRef] [PubMed]

Eisenberg, N., Fabes, R. A., & Spinrad, T. L. (2006). Prosocial behavior. In N. Eisenberg, W. Damon, & R. M. Lerner (Eds.), *Handbook of child psychology: Social, emotional, and personality development* (6th ed., Vol. 3, pp. 646–718). Wiley.

Elgar, F. J., Napoletano, A., Saul, G., Dirks, M. A., Craig, W., Poteat, V. P., & Koenig, B. W. (2014). Cyberbullying victimization and mental health in adolescents and the moderating role of family dinners. *JAMA Pediatrics, 168*(11), 1015–1022. [CrossRef] [PubMed]

Fabris, M. A., Badenes-Ribera, L., & Longobardi, C. (2021). Bullying victimization and muscle dysmorphic disorder in Italian adolescents: The mediating role of attachment to peers. *Children and Youth Services Review, 120*, 105720. [CrossRef]

Fabris, M. A., Longobardi, C., Morese, R., & Marengo, D. (2022). Exploring multivariate profiles of psychological distress and empathy in early adolescent victims, bullies, and bystanders involved in cyberbullying episodes. *International Journal of Environmental Research and Public Health, 19*(16), 9871. [CrossRef]

Fabris, M. A., Settanni, M., Longobardi, C., & Marengo, D. (2023). Sense of belonging at school and on social media in adolescence: Associations with educational achievement and psychosocial maladjustment. *Child Psychiatry & Human Development, 55*, 1620–1633. [CrossRef]

Fisher, B. W., Gardella, J. H., & Teurbe-Tolon, A. R. (2016). Peer cybervictimization among adolescents and the associated internalizing and externalizing problems: A meta-analysis. *Journal of Youth and Adolescence, 45*, 1727–1743. [CrossRef]

Fu, X., Li, S., Shen, C., Zhu, K., Zhang, M., Liu, Y., & Zhang, M. (2023). Effect of prosocial behavior on school bullying victimization among children and adolescents: Peer and student–teacher relationships as mediators. *Journal of Adolescence, 95*(2), 322–335. [CrossRef]

Gallego-Jiménez, M. G., & Rodríguez Otero, L. M. (2025). Adicción a internet y ciberbullying en alumnado español de formación profesional. *Health and Addictions/Salud y Drogas, 25*(1), 54–67. [CrossRef]

Gardella, J. H., Fisher, B. W., & Teurbe-Tolon, A. R. (2017). A systematic review and meta-analysis of cyber-victimization and educational outcomes for adolescents. *Review of Educational Research, 87*(2), 283–308. [CrossRef]

Geng, J., Bao, L., Wang, J., Wei, X., Zeng, P., & Lei, L. (2022). The maladaptive side of Internet altruists: Relationship between Internet altruistic behavior and cyberbullying victimization. *Children and Youth Services Review, 134*, 106362. [CrossRef]

Ginanjar, Y. E., Yahya, M., & Samana, A. (2024). Development of an integrative learning model for character education based on islamic values of the koran and hadith in boarding school. *Journal of Multidisciplinary Academic and Practice Studies, 2*(2), 147–167. [CrossRef]

Gini, G., Card, N. A., & Pozzoli, T. (2018). A meta-analysis of the differential relations of traditional and cyber-victimization with internalizing problems. *Aggressive Behavior, 44*(2), 185–198. [CrossRef] [PubMed]

Goodman, A., Lamping, D. L., & Ploubidis, G. B. (2010). When to use broader internalising and externalising subscales instead of the hypothesised five subscales on the Strengths and Difficulties Questionnaire (SDQ): Data from British parents, teachers and children. *Journal of Abnormal Child Psychology, 38*(8), 1179–1191. [CrossRef] [PubMed]

Goodman, R. (1997). The Strengths and Difficulties Questionnaire: A research note. *Journal of Child Psychology and Psychiatry, 38*, 581–586. [CrossRef]

Hellström, L., Thornberg, R., & Espelage, D. L. (2021). Definitions of bullying. In *The Wiley Blackwell handbook of bullying: A comprehensive and international review of research and intervention* (Vol. 1, pp. 2–21). John Wiley & Sons.

Holfeld, B., & Mishna, F. (2019). Internalizing symptoms and externalizing problems: Risk factors for or consequences of cyber victimization? *Journal of Youth and Adolescence, 48*, 567–580. [CrossRef]

Jadambaa, A., Thomas, H. J., Scott, J. G., Graves, N., Brain, D., & Pacella, R. (2019). Prevalence of traditional bullying and cyberbullying among children and adolescents in Australia: A systematic review and meta-analysis. *Australian & New Zealand Journal of Psychiatry*, *53*(9), 878–888. [CrossRef]

Kaiser, S., Kyrrestad, H., & Fossum, S. (2020). Cyberbullying status and mental health in Norwegian adolescents. *Scandinavian Journal of Psychology*, *61*(5), 707–713. [CrossRef]

Keith, S., Scheuerman, H. L., & Smith, A. L. (2025). Going viral: Investigating the short-and long-term traumatic effects of cyberbullying victimization on adolescents in schools. *Psychological Trauma: Theory, Research, Practice, and Policy*. [CrossRef]

Kokkinos, C. M., & Kipritsi, E. (2012). The relationship between bullying, victimization, trait emotional intelligence, self-efficacy and empathy among preadolescents. *Social Psychology of Education*, *15*, 41–58. [CrossRef]

Lee, J. Y., Chung, I. J., & Miller, D. B. (2022). The developmental trajectories of prosocial behavior in adolescence: A growth-mixture model. *Child Indicators Research*, *15*(1), 161–178. [CrossRef]

Li, C., Wang, P., Martin-Moratinos, M., Bella-Fernández, M., & Blasco-Fontecilla, H. (2024). Traditional bullying and cyberbullying in the digital age and its associated mental health problems in children and adolescents: A meta-analysis. *European Child & Adolescent Psychiatry*, *33*(9), 2895–2909. [CrossRef]

Lin, S., Longobardi, C., Fabris, M. A., & Settanni, M. (2025). Being kicked out of a WhatsApp group: Frequency and association with adolescents' psychosocial well-being and School Achievement. *Journal of Social and Personal Relationships*, *42*(1), 318–336. [CrossRef]

Lin, S., Longobardi, C., Mastrokoukou, S., & Fabris, M. A. (2024). Bullying victimization and psychological adjustment in Chinese students: The mediating role of teacher–student relationships. *School Psychology International*, *46*(1), 68–89. [CrossRef]

Longobardi, C., Badenes-Ribera, L., Fabris, M. A., Martinez, A., & McMahon, S. D. (2019a). Prevalence of student violence against teachers: A meta-analysis. *Psychology of Violence*, *9*(6), 596. [CrossRef]

Longobardi, C., Morese, R., & Fabris, M. A. (2020). COVID-19 emergency: Social distancing and social exclusion as risks for suicide ideation and attempts in adolescents. *Frontiers in Psychology*, *11*, 551113. [CrossRef]

Longobardi, C., Prino, L. E., Fabris, M. A., & Settanni, M. (2017). School violence in two Mediterranean countries: Italy and Albania. *Children and Youth Services Review*, *82*, 254–261. [CrossRef]

Longobardi, C., Prino, L. E., Fabris, M. A., & Settanni, M. (2019b). Violence in school: An investigation of physical, psychological, and sexual victimization reported by Italian adolescents. *Journal of School Violence*, *18*(1), 49–61. [CrossRef]

Longobardi, C., Settanni, M., Lin, S., & Fabris, M. A. (2021). Student–teacher relationship quality and prosocial behaviour: The mediating role of academic achievement and a positive attitude towards school. *British Journal of Educational Psychology*, *91*(2), 547–562. [CrossRef]

Marciano, L., Schulz, P. J., & Camerini, A. L. (2020). Cyberbullying perpetration and victimization in youth: A meta-analysis of longitudinal studies. *Journal of Computer-Mediated Communication*, *25*(2), 163–181. [CrossRef]

Marengo, D., Jungert, T., Iotti, N. O., Settanni, M., Thornberg, R., & Longobardi, C. (2018). Conflictual student–teacher relationship, emotional and behavioral problems, prosocial behavior, and their associations with bullies, victims, and bullies/victims. *Educational Psychology*, *38*(9), 1201–1217. [CrossRef]

Marengo, D., Settanni, M., Fabris, M. A., & Longobardi, C. (2021). Alone, together: Fear of missing out mediates the link between peer exclusion in WhatsApp classmate groups and psychological adjustment in early-adolescent teens. *Journal of Social and Personal Relationships*, *38*(4), 1371–1379. [CrossRef]

Marengo, D., Settanni, M., Mastrokoukou, S., Fabris, M. A., & Longobardi, C. (2024). Social Media Linked to early adolescent suicidal thoughts via cyberbullying and internalizing symptoms. *International Journal of Bullying Prevention*, 1–10. [CrossRef]

Marsh, H. W., Lüdtke, O., Trautwein, U., & Morin, A. J. S. (2009). Classical latent profile analysis of academic self-concept dimensions: Synergy of person-and variable-centered approaches to theoretical models of self-concept. *Structural Equation Modeling: A Multidisciplinary Journal*, *16*(2), 191–225. [CrossRef]

Modecki, K. L., Minchin, J., Harbaugh, A. G., Guerra, N. G., & Runions, K. C. (2014). Bullying prevalence across contexts: A meta-analysis measuring cyber and traditional bullying. *Journal of Adolescent Health*, *55*(5), 602–611. [CrossRef] [PubMed]

Moore, S. E., Norman, R. E., Suetani, S., Thomas, H. J., Sly, P. D., & Scott, J. G. (2017). Consequences of bullying victimization in childhood and adolescence: A systematic review and meta-analysis. *World Journal of Psychiatry*, *7*(1), 60. [CrossRef]

Morese, R., Fabris, M. A., Longobardi, C., & Marengo, D. (2024). Involvement in cyberbullying events and empathy are related to emotional responses to simulated social pain tasks. *Digital Health*, *10*, 20552076241253085. [CrossRef]

Nylund-Gibson, K., & Choi, A. Y. (2018). Ten frequently asked questions about latent class analysis. *Translational Issues in Psychological Science*, *4*(4), 440–461. [CrossRef]

Ossa, F. C., Jantzer, V., Neumayer, F., Eppelmann, L., Resch, F., & Kaess, M. (2023). Cyberbullying and school bullying are related to additive adverse effects among adolescents. *Psychopathology*, *56*(1–2), 127–137. [CrossRef]

Parada, R. (2000). *Adolescent peer relations instrument: A theoretical and empirical basis for the measurement of participant roles in bullying and victimisation of adolescence: An interim test manual and a research monograph: A test manual*. Publication Unit, Self-concept Enhancement and Learning Facilitation (SELF) Research Centre, University of Western Sydney.

Pengpid, S., & Peltzer, K. (2023). Combined victimization of face-to-face and cyberbullying and adverse health outcomes among school-age adolescents in Argentina. *Psychology, Health & Medicine*, *28*(8), 2261–2272. [CrossRef]

Prino, L. E., Longobardi, C., Fabris, M. A., Parada, R. H., & Settanni, M. (2019). Effects of bullying victimization on internalizing and externalizing symptoms: The mediating role of alexithymia. *Journal of Child and Family Studies*, *28*, 2586–2593. [CrossRef]

Ran, H., Yang, Q., Fang, D., Che, Y., Chen, L., Liang, X., Sun, H., Peng, J., Wang, S., & Xiao, Y. (2023). Social indicators with serious injury and school bullying victimization in vulnerable adolescents aged 12–15 years: Data from the Global School-Based Student Survey. *Journal of affective disorders*, *324*, 469–476. [CrossRef] [PubMed]

Reinecke, J. (2006). Longitudinal Analysis of Adolescents' Deviant and Delinquent Behavior. *Methodology*, *2*(3), 100–112. [CrossRef]

Rostam-Abadi, Y., Stefanovics, E. A., & Potenza, M. N. (2024). An exploratory study of the prevalence and adverse associations of in-school traditional bullying and cyberbullying among adolescents in Connecticut. *Journal of Psychiatric Research*, *173*, 372–380. [CrossRef] [PubMed]

Saleem, S., Khan, N. F., Zafar, S., & Ahmed, M. (2025). Cyberbullying victimization among university students—A national study of Pakistan. *Security Journal*, *38*(1), 23. [CrossRef]

Samara, M., Da Silva Nascimento, B., El-Asam, A., Hammuda, S., & Khattab, N. (2021). How can bullying victimisation lead to lower academic achievement? A systematic review and meta-analysis of the mediating role of cognitive-motivational factors. *International Journal of Environmental Research and Public Health*, *18*(5), 2209. [CrossRef]

Schneider, S. K., O'donnell, L., Stueve, A., & Coulter, R. W. (2012). Cyberbullying, school bullying, and psychological distress: A regional census of high school students. *American Journal of Public Health*, *102*(1), 171–177. [CrossRef]

Shahrour, G., Dardas, L. A., Al-Khayat, A., & Al-Qasem, A. (2020). Prevalence, correlates, and experiences of school bullying among adolescents: A national study in Jordan. *School Psychology International*, *41*(5), 430–453. [CrossRef]

Sobol, M., Przepiórka, A., & Błachnio, A. (2025). Factors contributing to the defending behavior of adolescent cyberbystanders: A systematic review and meta-analysis. *Computers in Human Behavior*, *162*, 108463. [CrossRef]

Thomas, H. J., Connor, J. P., & Scott, J. G. (2015). Integrating traditional bullying and cyberbullying: Challenges of definition and measurement in adolescents—A review. *Educational Psychology Review*, *27*, 135–152. [CrossRef]

Thomas, K. J., & McCuddy, T. (2020). Affinity, affiliation, and guilt: Examining between-and within-person variability in delinquent peer influence. *Justice Quarterly*, *37*(4), 715–738. [CrossRef]

Thornton, E., Panayiotou, M., & Humphrey, N. (2024). Prevalence, inequalities, and impact of bullying in adolescence: Insights from the# BeeWell study. *International Journal of Bullying Prevention*, 1–19. [CrossRef]

Topcu, Ç., & Erdur-Baker, Ö. (2018). RCBI-II: The second revision of the revised cyber bullying inventory. *Measurement and Evaluation in Counseling and Development*, *51*(1), 32–41. [CrossRef]

Valente, J. Y., Ferreira-Junior, V., Paiva de Oliveira Galvão, P., de la Torre, A., & Sanchez, Z. M. (2024). Psychiatric symptoms as predictors of latent classes of bullying victimization and perpetration among early adolescents. *Current Psychology*, *43*(1), 204–213. [CrossRef]

Völlink, T., Bolman, C. A., Dehue, F., & Jacobs, N. C. (2013). Coping with cyberbullying: Differences between victims, bully-victims and children not involved in bullying. *Journal of Community & Applied Social Psychology*, *23*(1), 7–24.

Wang, C., Li, B., Zhang, L., Liu, Y., & Xu, P. (2024). Prosocial behavior and teachers' attitudes towards bullying on peer victimization among middle school students: Examining the cross-level moderating effect of classroom climate. *School Psychology Review*, *53*(5), 579–592. [CrossRef]

Wang, Z., Cheng, L., Xie, Z., & Jiang, C. (2024). Cyberbullying victimization and perpetration: The influence on cyberostracism and youth anxiety. *Behavioral Sciences & the Law*, *42*(4), 461–473. [CrossRef]

Wright, M. F. (2015). Adolescents' cyber aggression perpetration and cyber victimization: The longitudinal associations with school functioning. *Social Psychology of Education*, *18*, 653–666. [CrossRef]

European Journal of
Investigation in Health, Psychology and Education

MDPI

Article

Examining the Impact of a Behavior Modification Program on Disease Prevention Behaviors among Individuals at Risk of Diabetes: A Quasi-Experimental Investigation

Thanatkorn Phudphad [1], Supat Teravecharoenchai [1,*], Panit Khemtong [1] and Wanich Suksatan [1,2,*]

[1] Department of Public Health, Faculty of Liberal Arts, Krirk University, Bangkok 10220, Thailand; kornthanatkorn@gmail.com (T.P.); fedupnk@ku.ac.th (P.K.)
[2] Midwest Health Professionals, Saint Louis, MO 63119, USA
* Correspondence: supat.kru@gmail.com (S.T.); wanich.suk@hotmail.com (W.S.)

Abstract: This study aimed to develop and test a behavior modification intervention to prevent type 2 diabetes (T2DM) among at-risk individuals. The primary goal was to compare diabetes prevention behaviors and fasting blood sugar levels between the intervention and comparison groups. This study utilizes a quasi-experimental design to develop a behavior modification intervention for preventing diabetes. It involves two groups, each with pre- and post-intervention assessments, comprising 60 at-risk individuals equally divided into intervention and comparison groups. The 8-week intervention includes components like risk assessment, dietary skill enhancement, exercise, stress management, and social media platforms (data recording training, follow-up visits, reminders, and visual aids). Data collection includes self-administered questionnaires and blood sugar level measurements. Statistical analysis involved paired *t*-tests for within-group comparisons and independent *t*-tests for between-group differences. The findings showed that the intervention group achieved significantly higher average scores in nutrition, exercise, and stress management, and had significantly lower average blood sugar levels compared to the comparison group. These results suggest that healthcare providers and policymakers should develop community health programs and public health policies that incorporate integrative care, leverage social media platforms, and foster collaboration with other health professionals to improve outcomes for individuals at risk of T2DM.

Keywords: behavior modification intervention; blood sugar levels; diabetes; exercise; health behaviors; social media; type 2 diabetes prevention

1. Introduction

Type 2 diabetes mellitus (T2DM), a chronic non-communicable disease, currently represents a significant global public health challenge, with its prevalence steadily increasing each year [1]. There were 537 million individuals diagnosed with diabetes worldwide in 2021, a figure projected to rise to 643 million by 2030 and 783 million by 2045 [2]. In the Pacific region, as of 2017, Thailand reported 6.1 million individuals with diabetes, ranking fourth after China, Indonesia, and Japan [2]. The incidence of diabetes in Thailand is continually rising, with an estimated 300,000 new cases annually and 3.2 million individuals currently registered in the Ministry of Public Health's system. Global health expenditure related to diabetes was estimated to be USD 966 billion in 2021 and is projected to increase to USD 1045 billion by 2045 [1]. Moreover, diabetes remains a primary contributor to the onset of various other non-communicable diseases (NCDs), including heart disease, stroke, hypertension, and kidney disease [3].

Given the incurable nature of diabetes and its potential for genetic transmission, prevention in individuals at risk is more crucial than ever. The long latency period before symptoms appear causes many at-risk individuals to remain unaware and fail to manage their condition early on [4]. Although the Ministry of Public Health of Thailand has implemented the Chronic Care Model as a guideline for managing care for people at risk for diabetes, it has been found that the results still lack consistency in practice as a model to promote concrete behavior change [5]. Consequently, the number of at-risk individuals and diabetic patients continues to rise [6].

The increasing trend in T2DM represents a significant public health problem that requires urgent intervention to reduce future incidence rates [7,8]. The most effective way to control and prevent diabetes is through lifestyle changes, particularly for those at risk. Emphasizing the prevention of diabetes development in high-risk groups is crucial, as individuals at high risk can delay or even avoid the onset of the disease by modifying their lifestyle behaviors (therapeutic lifestyle changes) [9]. Early detection and lifestyle interventions, such as regular physical activity, choosing appropriate foods, consuming vegetables and fruits high in fiber, and avoiding sweet, fatty, and salty foods, are essential [10]. Additionally, learning to manage stress and maintaining a positive outlook can significantly reduce the incidence of diabetes [11].

A comprehensive review of the literature and previous research on behavior modification programs for individuals at risk for diabetes and T2DM populations, both in Thailand [12–14] and internationally [15–17], indicates that foreign countries employ a diverse array of health behavior modification programs. These programs aim to impart self-management knowledge and elevate awareness regarding personal healthcare. In similar contexts, the effects of behavior modification programs on the exercise behavior of high-risk individuals with T2DM have shown that the average exercise behavior score of the intervention group was significantly higher than that of the comparison group after the experiment [13,14,18]. The findings from these studies suggest that the most effective strategy to address T2DM involves preventing its onset in at-risk groups by enhancing their knowledge and perceptions, thereby promoting positive changes in self-care behaviors [6].

In the context of Ratchaburi Province, Thailand, there is a notably high rate of diabetes patients. The rate of diabetes per 100,000 people for the fiscal years 2019, 2020, and 2021 is 638.15, 585.04, and 596.68, respectively. These figures indicate a likely increase in the rate of new diabetes cases per 100,000 people [19]. Additionally, Mueang Ratchaburi District, the fifth most populous subdistrict in Ratchaburi Province, has been actively screening for diabetes risk groups. Reports summarizing the results of diabetes risk screenings for individuals aged 35 years and over from fiscal years 2019 to 2021 indicate a continuous increase in the number of people at risk, with percentages of 0.81%, 33.43%, and 45.91%, respectively [19].

In response to this trend, we have developed a behavior modification model to prevent diabetes in groups at risk for T2DM, utilizing the Model of Self-Regulation to design activity plans that facilitate appropriate health behavior changes in these at-risk groups. The Model of Self-Regulation suggests that individuals' perceptions of their illness influence their coping strategies, which in turn affect health outcomes like glycemic control and quality of life [20]. Key components of this model include illness perceptions, general coping strategies, and specific strategies like adherence to treatment and health behaviors. These elements are essential for sustaining behavior changes and have been incorporated into our behavior modification model developed in this study.

Furthermore, we have incorporated the use of the LINE application to transmit health knowledge and enhance self-care skills related to diet, exercise, stress management, and problem-solving. This includes interactive video calls and sending LINE stickers to provide reminders and follow-ups, which are as effective as home visits and suitable for the current context, where the use of remote media has increased [21,22]. Therefore, this study aims to develop a behavior modification model to prevent diabetes in individuals with T2DM, and these outcomes were assessed before and after the program implementation. This approach is particularly beneficial in the COVID-19 situation, where social distancing reduces the need for home visits and hospital visits, allowing for continuous communication with the health team to address problems.

2. Materials and Methods

2.1. Research Design

This research employed a quasi-experimental design to evaluate the effectiveness of a behavior modification model for preventing diabetes in high-risk groups. This design was chosen due to several key factors and offers a practical and robust framework for evaluating the effectiveness of our behavior modification program, providing insights that are both applicable and actionable in real-world public health settings.

2.2. Setting and Participants

The participants of this study were individuals at risk of diabetes from Mueang Ratchaburi District, Ratchaburi Province, Thailand. The inclusion criteria for the sample group were as follows: individuals at risk for diabetes, both male and female, aged 35 years and above, proficient in reading, writing, and understanding Thai, possessing a smartphone, having a blood sugar level (DTX) of 100–125 mg/dL, being capable of exercise and self-care, and willing to participate in the modification program. Exclusion criteria included a diagnosis of diabetes by a physician, pregnancy, the presence of congenital diseases requiring continuous medication, relocation, requesting withdrawal from the study, or incomplete participation in the study.

The sample size for this study was determined using the G*Power 3.1 program [23]. An alpha significance level was set at 0.05 ($\alpha = 0.05$), with a power of 0.80 and an effect size of 0.80 [24], resulting in a required sample size of 27 participants per group. To account for potential dropouts, the sample size was increased by 15%, resulting in 30 participants per group. Consequently, the total sample size was 60 participants, divided into two groups, the intervention group and the comparison group, matched to have similar characteristics (matched pair). This study was conducted from September to December 2022.

2.3. Research Instruments

The three research instruments utilized to collect data were as follows:

Sociodemographic Data Form: This form consists of multiple-choice and fill-in-the-blank questions covering gender, age, marital status, education level, occupation, sufficiency of income, alcohol consumption, smoking, and receipt of information about diabetes.

Diabetes Prevention Behavior Scale (DPBS): Developed by the researchers through a review of the relevant literature and the Model of Self-Regulation [20], this scale comprises 57 questions divided into three areas: nutrition (30 questions), exercise (17 questions), and stress management (10 questions). For example, one question asks, "Do you read nutrition labels before purchasing food?" The scale employs a 5-level rating system: 1 = never practicing, 2 = rarely practicing, 3 = sometimes practicing, 4 = practicing almost every time, and 5 = practicing regularly. The criteria for interpreting diabetes prevention behavior are as follows: minimal (mean score 1.00–1.50), little (mean score 1.51–2.50), moderate (mean score 2.51–3.50), very high (mean score 3.51–4.50), and highest (mean score 4.51–5.00). This tool was examined by five qualified experts who tested for validity and item-objective congruence (IOC). Validities of nutrition, exercise, and stress management were 0.94, 0.96, and 0.92, respectively. The reliability of this instrument was tried out with 30 samples by finding Cronbach's alpha coefficient (α–coefficient), which equaled 0.94. The Cronbach's alpha coefficients in each component were as follows: nutrition questionnaires = 0.92, exercise questionnaire = 0.94, and stress management questionnaires = 0.96.

Health Record Form: This form includes open-ended questions and sections for recording health data and blood sugar levels (Dextrostix: DTX) from fingertip measurements taken after fasting for at least six hours, at two different times. The criteria for interpreting blood sugar levels are as follows [25]: normal ($<$100 mg/dL), at risk of diabetes (100–125 mg/dL), and diabetes ($\geq$126 mg/dL).

2.4. Data Collection

After receiving ethics approval from the research committees, the research team held a meeting to determine the scope of the research and the tools to be used. The researchers coordinated with the Subdistrict Health Promoting Hospital to request permission to collect data, clarifying the objectives and steps involved in conducting the research. The intervention procedure involved a study of the results of the prevention model for type 2 diabetes in individuals at risk. The researchers explained the participation process and obtained signed consent from the participants before implementing the modification model to prevent diabetes in the intervention group. There was no dropout in this study because we used the LINE application, including LINE stickers and messages, to maintain consistent communication with participants. This included sending reminders, motivational messages, and educational content related to diet, exercise, and stress management. Participants received individualized feedback based on their progress, which was designed to be constructive and encouraging, helping them to understand their achievements and areas for improvement. Additionally, we worked with participants to set realistic and achievable goals. Regularly reviewing and adjusting these goals helped maintain their motivation and adherence to the program. Conducted between September and December 2022, the program lasted 8 weeks and included the following activities:

Intervention Group:

Week 1:

- Evaluate diabetes prevention behavior and sugar levels before the experiment (pre-test).
- Organize activities at the Subdistrict Health Promoting Hospital, starting with relationship building and providing knowledge about diabetes. The intervention group participated in self-assessment of their diabetes risk. Activities included learning about eating, exercising, and managing emotions/stress through three activity stations. Participants wrote down goals to achieve within the two months of the program, practiced recording daily information via Google Forms, and set up a LINE group for behavior change communication and sending reminder stickers.

Week 2:

- Organize activities at the Subdistrict Health Promoting Hospital to review knowledge and exchange experiences using models of at-risk individuals with good self-care practices. Small groups were formed to encourage and remind each other to practice daily diabetes prevention behaviors. Group discussions addressed problems and obstacles in practice.
- The intervention group practiced daily diabetes prevention activities and sent information via Google Forms. Encouragement and praise were provided through the LINE group.

Week 3:

- Organize home visits at designated meeting points to exchange experiences, solve problems, and boost morale. Review training on eating, exercise, and emotional management skills for the intervention group to practice daily diabetes prevention behaviors; information sent via Google Forms. Encouragement and praise continued through the LINE group.
- Follow-up visits by phone/LINE to monitor progress, address obstacles, and provide encouragement.

Week 4:

- Organize home visits at designated meeting points to exchange experiences, solve obstacles, and strengthen morale. Review training on eating, exercise, and emotional management skills for the intervention group to practice daily diabetes prevention behaviors; information sent via Google Forms. Encouragement and praise continued through the LINE group.

- Follow-up visits by phone/LINE to monitor progress, address obstacles, and provide encouragement.

Weeks 5–7:

- Organize activities at the Subdistrict Health Promoting Hospital to exchange experiences, solve obstacles, and strengthen morale. Review eating, exercise, and emotional management practices for the intervention group to practice daily diabetes prevention behaviors and send information via Google Forms. Encouragement and praise continued through the LINE group.
- Follow-up visits by phone/LINE to monitor progress, address obstacles, and provide encouragement.

Week 8:

- Organize activities at the Subdistrict Health Promoting Hospital to summarize the results of the activities, provide words of encouragement to the intervention group, and make a commitment to continue correct and sustainable behaviors. Evaluate diabetes prevention behavior and blood sugar levels after the experiment (post-test).

Comparison Group:

Week 1: Personal information and diabetes prevention behavior questionnaires were collected at the Subdistrict Health Promoting Hospital, which took 15–20 min. Participants received 5–10 min of individual general advice on self-care for diabetes and were advised as needed if they had questions.
Weeks 2–7: Participants in the comparison group took care of themselves at home as usual.
Week 8: The researchers repeated the data collection. After completing data collection, the researchers offered an 8-week behavior modification program on disease prevention behaviors to the comparison group.

2.5. Data Analysis

The Statistical Package for Social Sciences (SPSS) version 25.0 software was employed for data analysis. Descriptive statistics, including percentages, means, and standard deviations, were used to analyze general data. The normality of the data distribution was assessed using the Kolmogorov–Smirnov test. Independent t-tests were utilized to compare the mean scores for nutrition behavior, exercise, stress management, and blood sugar levels between the intervention and comparison groups post-intervention. Paired t-tests were conducted to assess differences in mean scores for food consumption behavior, exercise, mood management, and blood sugar levels before and after the intervention within the intervention group. Statistical significance was determined at the 0.05 level (p-value <0.05).

3. Results

In this study, the intervention and comparison group samples of 60 people had similar characteristics. In the intervention group, the average age was 57.8 years (S.D. = 9.72). The majority were married (70.0%), had a lower primary education level (40.0%), and were generally employed (40.0%). The average monthly income was USD 185.19 (S.D. = 160.04), with 57.1% having enough income to save, 86.7% not drinking alcohol, and 100% not smoking.

In the comparison group, the average age was 51.6 years (S.D. = 5.28). Most were married (56.7%), had a lower primary education level (43.3%), and were occupied with housework (33.3%). The average monthly income was USD 189.52 (S.D. = 125.29), with 53.3% having sufficient income but not enough to save, 96.7% not drinking alcohol, and 100% not smoking, as shown in Table 1.

Table 1. Sociodemographic characteristics of the participants.

Demographic Characteristics	Intervention Group		Comparison Group		Total	
	N	%	N	%	N	%
Sex						
Female	30	100.0	29	96.70	59	98.30
Male	0	0.00	1	3.30	1	1.10
Age (years)	Mean ± SD = 57.8 ± 9.72		Mean ± SD = 58.1 ± 11.87		Mean ± SD = 58.04 ± 10.80	
35–40	1	3.30	2	6.60	3	5.00
41–50	7	23.40	4	13.30	11	18.30
51–60	9	30.00	9	30.00	18	30.00
61–70	9	30.00	9	36.70	20	33.30
>70	4	13.30	4	13.30	8	13.40
Marital status						
Single	2	6.70	3	10.00	5	8.30
Married	21	70.00	17	56.70	38	63.30
Divorced/Windowed	7	23.40	10	33.40	17	28.40
Education level						
Primary school	19	63.30	20	66.60	39	65.10
High school or higher	11	36.60	10	33.30	21	34.90
Current Occupation						
Agriculturist	5	16.70	4	13.30	9	15.00
Businessperson/trade	5	16.70	8	26.70	13	21.60
Employment	12	40.0	8	26.70	20	33.40
Unemployment/retired	8	26.7	10	33.30	18	30.00
Income (USD)	Mean ± SD = 185.19 ± 160.04		Mean ± SD = 189.52 ± 125.29		Mean ± SD = 174.69 ± 142.97	
<140	16	57.1	16	53.3	32	53.4
141–285	10	35.8	10	33.4	20	33.3
>286–430	2	6.60	4	13.30	6	10.00
Prefer not to answer	2	6.60	0	0.00	2	3.30
Income sufficiency						
Sufficient and saving	3	10.00	6	20.00	9	15.00
Sufficient without saving	19	53.30	18	60.00	37	61.70
Insufficient	6	30.00	6	20.00	12	20.00
Prefer not to answer	2	6.700	0	0.00	2	3.30
Alcohol drinking history						
Drinking	2	6.70	1	3.30	3	5.00
No drinking	26	86.70	29	96.70	55	91.70
Quit drinking	2	6.70	0	0.00	2	3.30
Smoking history						
No smoking	30	100.00	30	100.00	60	100.00
Received information about T2DM						
Received	29	96.7	27	90.0	56	93.3
No Received	1	3.3	3	10.0	4	6.7

Notes: SD = standard deviation, T2DM = type 2 diabetes mellitus.

After participating in the behavior modification program, the intervention group exhibited higher diabetes prevention behaviors in each component and overall compared to before the program. These behaviors were significantly more pronounced than those of the comparison group. The results of comparing the mean values of diabetes prevention behaviors revealed that after participating in the program, the intervention group demonstrated higher diabetes prevention behaviors than before the intervention and significantly higher than the comparison group. Additionally, it was found that the mean blood sugar levels after abstaining from food for 6 h were lower in the intervention group after participating in the program compared to before the program, and significantly lower than those of the comparison group, as shown in Table 2.

Table 2. Outcome of a behavior modification program on disease prevention behaviors among individuals at risk of diabetes.

Variables	Intervention Group		Comparison Group		t	p-Value
	Mean ± SD	Interpretation	Mean ± SD	Interpretation		
Diabetes Prevention Behaviors					14.13	<0.01
Before	2.81 ± 0.37	Moderate	3.10 ± 0.38	Moderate		
After	4.09 ± 0.39	Good	2.94 ± 0.21	Moderate		
Nutrition					11.57	<0.01
Before	2.38 ± 0.32	Fair	3.26 ± 0.32	Moderate		
After	3.91 ± 0.30	Good	3.10 ± 0.23	Moderate		
Exercise					11.68	<0.01
Before	2.45 ± 0.62	Fair	2.55 ± 0.84	Moderate		
After	4.24 ± 0.73	Good	2.39 ± 0.46	Fair		
Stress management					8.31	<0.01
Before	3.31 ± 0.51	Moderate	3.55 ± 0.39	Good		
After	4.38 ± 0.44	Good	3.41 ± 0.46	Moderate		
Blood sugar level					−1.962	0.05
Before	120.96 ± 24.48	Risk of Diabetes	108.80 ± 19.68	Risk of Diabetes		
After	98.63 ± 13.35	Normal	108.03 ± 22.58	Risk of Diabetes		

4. Discussion

The results of this study indicated that the intervention group, after participating in the program, exhibited better overall diabetes prevention behaviors, including each component and blood sugar levels, compared to before participating in the program and significantly better than the comparison group. This improvement can be attributed to the behavior modification model to prevent diabetes, which included demonstrations and practice sessions. The intervention group was able to observe successful behavior modification experiences for diabetes prevention. Practicing eating and exercise habits after the demonstrations allowed the intervention group to achieve their own successes. The program also involved monitoring and supporting activities through a self-directed program combined with the LINE application. The Model of Self-Regulation, based on the Kanfer and Hagerman [20] concept, posits that a person's behavior cannot be changed by anyone other than themselves and that behavior change relies on motivation, leading individuals to accept and recognize the benefits of such change.

In this study, it was found that most of the intervention group were motivated to engage in the activities because they wanted to avoid suffering from chronic diseases. The intervention group recognized the benefits of dietary changes, exercise, and stress management. Activities included setting weight loss goals to reduce the risk of developing diabetes due to behavioral factors. Participants in the intervention group were asked to analyze the causes of being overweight and their inability to control their weight, and then set short-term and long-term goals that matched their needs. The intervention group received training in various skills, including calculating energy and food portions for each meal, selecting food exchange menus, practicing belly rubbing on a chair, breath-holding practice (prana training), and receiving pamphlets on diabetes prevention to take home and review. This training enabled the participants to understand and accurately implement these practices [15]. They were encouraged to self-regulate by recording their daily food intake, exercise frequency, and stress management each week using Google Forms. Additionally, they conducted self-assessments by comparing their body weight data with their set goals. The experiment found that those who consistently lost weight saw better results, recognized the benefits of the activities, and were motivated to continue participating in the activities.

For cases in the intervention group where the results did not meet the goals, participants received reinforcement and adjusted their goals accordingly. Additionally, the intervention group received support from members of a LINE group established for communication. This group shared various information in the form of text, images, video clips, and stickers. For example, they posted pictures of daily meals to aid weight loss and exercise clips from each team to encourage and follow and provided opportunities to ask questions and give suggestions. The use of the LINE application for communication allowed the intervention group to talk, exchange information, provide reminders, and ask questions about any problems they encountered while performing activities [21]. This constant communication ensured that the intervention group received accurate information, had confidence in continuing their behaviors, and felt encouraged to keep participating in the activities. In addition to verbal praise from LINE group members, messages and stickers were sent to reinforce positive behaviors [26]. In this study, the researcher team supported participants by making home visits and follow-up phone calls to assess the self-regulation progress of the intervention group. This consistent reinforcement helped the intervention group maintain their behaviors throughout the 8-week program, resulting in significant improvements in their eating, exercising, and stress management behaviors.

From the above information, it can be seen that the intervention group improved their eating behavior by controlling food portions according to the specified energy guidelines and developed better eating habits. Weighing themselves weekly and observing weight loss provided encouragement to continue self-regulation and also reminded their partners to self-regulate according to their goals. This is consistent with previous studies [13,14,18], which examined the effects of a self-regulation program on food consumption behaviors in individuals at high risk for diabetes. The results indicated that after participating in the program, the intervention group had significantly higher mean food consumption behaviors compared to the comparison group, with statistical significance at the 0.05 level. Our findings are also consistent with the study in Spain [27], which investigated the effects of a Spanish diabetes self-management program to promote self-efficacy in changing food consumption behavior in individuals with T2DM based on self-efficacy theory. After the experiment, the intervention group showed increases in average scores for self-efficacy in each component, diet, physical activity, and disease control, ranging from 0.5 (95% CI: 0.1 to 0.9) to 0.8 (95% CI: 0.5 to 1.2) [27]. Furthermore, our study aligns with the findings of a meta-analysis from 30 meta-analyses published between 2007 and 2017 aggregating data from 409,185 participants [28]. Their research indicated that after receiving the interventions to promote healthy eating, the intervention groups exhibited better eating habits compared to the comparison group, with statistical significance [28].

In this study, the exercise behavior of the intervention group improved significantly after using the behavior modification model to prevent diabetes, transitioning from a low level to a high level. After the experiment, the intervention group showed an average increase in exercise behavior. This improvement was due to daily practice and self-regulation, with participants recording their exercise each day via Google Forms throughout the 8-week program. The findings of this study are consistent with previous studies in Thailand [13,18], which examined the effects of a self-regulation program on the exercise behavior of high-risk individuals with diabetes. The results indicated that, after the experiment, the average exercise behavior score of the intervention group was significantly higher than that of the comparison group ($p < 0.05$) [13]. Additionally, the results from a previous study showed that the diabetic risk group in the intervention group had a greater increase in the mean exercise behavior score than the comparison group ($p < 0.001$), with the mean score increasing by 0.75 points (95% CI: 0.49, 1.00) [18]. Furthermore, our study corroborates the findings of a previous study conducted in the United States, which demonstrated that the self-regulation strategies with the most significant increase in frequency over time included tracking physical activity, considering one's environment, rewarding oneself for engaging in physical activity, making physical activity more enjoyable, setting goals, and experimenting with different types of physical activity [28]. These changes were statistically significant at the $p < 0.001$ level.

In terms of stress management behavior, we found that the intervention group improved from a moderate to a high level after using the behavior modification model to prevent diabetes. Additionally, the intervention group had higher stress management behavior scores than before receiving the model, and they were higher than the comparison group. This can be explained by the model's inclusion of stress management techniques, such as meditation and breath-holding practice (prana training), demonstrated by the researchers. The program also facilitated an exchange of experiences within the group regarding stress management, enabling the intervention group to practice stress management independently. These findings are consistent with the studies in Thailand, which found that after participating in the empower home visiting program using a family tree, the sample group had a higher mean score for stress management and disease prevention behaviors than before participating in the program, with statistical significance at the 0.05 level (p-value <0.05) [29]. Clinical outcomes, including blood pressure levels, blood sugar levels, and body mass index, also improved significantly [29]. Similarly, the previous reviews investigated the effectiveness of a health behavior change program to improve adherence to chronic disease medications [30], showing that the intervention group developed stress management skills, resulting in positive perceptions of their experiences. Consequently, the intervention group was able to effectively manage stress [31].

The primary strength of the present study lies in its originality, as it is the first to develop a behavior modification model for individuals at risk of T2DM in rural communities by incorporating the use of the LINE application and Google Forms to transmit health knowledge and enhance self-care skills related to diet, exercise, stress management, and problem-solving. By applying self-regulation theory, the behavior modification model successfully facilitated behavioral changes in eating habits, exercise, and stress management, and led to improved blood sugar levels. These findings underscore the effectiveness of the behavior modification model in preventing T2DM, demonstrating its potential applicability to at-risk groups in similar contexts. The behavior modification model used in this study can be adapted to urban environments where access to healthcare facilities and technology might be more readily available. Urban areas often have diverse populations with varying levels of health literacy and access to resources. By tailoring the intervention to consider these factors, such as leveraging local community centers for in-person workshops or using mobile health (mHealth) technologies to reach a wider audience, the program can effectively address the needs of urban residents. The use of the LINE application in this study highlights the potential for digital tools to support health interventions. In urban and culturally diverse settings, similar platforms that are popular and widely used by the target population can be utilized to maintain communication, provide educational content, and support behavior change. This approach ensures that the intervention is accessible and relevant to the participants' daily lives. Additionally, to effectively implement and sustain T2DM prevention programs, healthcare providers and policymakers should develop comprehensive training and education modules, implement patient-centered care plans, and utilize technology for continuous engagement and monitoring. They should also establish standardized systems for tracking progress, allocate sufficient funding, and promote community-based interventions. Public awareness campaigns and cross-sector collaboration are crucial, along with integrating diabetes prevention into existing health programs and fostering international cooperation. These steps will enhance the effectiveness of T2DM prevention initiatives and improve health outcomes for at-risk populations.

The effectiveness of the behavior modification intervention to prevent T2DM among at-risk individuals can be significantly influenced by various cultural and contextual factors. Culturally, dietary habits and exercise norms in Thailand may differ from those in other countries, affecting how participants engage with dietary recommendations and physical activity guidelines [32]. For instance, traditional Thai diets rich in rice and certain fats might need specific adaptations in the intervention to align with healthy eating practices. Additionally, cultural beliefs about health and illness can shape participants' perceptions of T2DM prevention and their willingness to adopt recommended behaviors [3]. Finally, policy and environmental factors, such as government policies promoting healthy lifestyles and the physical environment's support for physical activity and healthy eating, can significantly impact the intervention's effectiveness. Supportive policies and a conducive environment can facilitate the adoption of healthy behaviors and sustain the intervention's benefits.

The present study has several limitations. First, the participants were individuals at risk of diabetes from only one province in Thailand, which may constrain the generalizability of our findings to other populations in different contexts, such as urban communities and nursing homes. Future studies should explore the application of this behavior modification model in various urban and cultural contexts to validate its adaptability and effectiveness. Comparative studies can help identify which modifications are most effective in different settings, further refining the model for broader application. Second, we utilized only the DTX method to assess blood glucose levels after fasting for at least 6–8 h. While this method is suitable for mass screening programs for individuals at risk of diabetes due to its accuracy and rapid results, future studies should employ other standard methods for evaluating blood glucose levels in individuals at risk of diabetes, such as fasting plasma glucose or HbA1c levels. Third, the current study focused on short-term outcomes, necessitating more in-depth investigation into the relationship between demographic data, health behaviors, and clinical outcomes. Future interventional studies should aim to clarify the long-term outcomes of individuals at risk of diabetes with extended interventions. To ensure the sustainability of the intervention, future research should explore ways to integrate it into routine healthcare practices. This might involve training healthcare providers to deliver the intervention during regular check-ups or incorporating it into community health programs. Scalability and adaptability studies are crucial to determine how the intervention can be expanded to larger populations and adapted to different cultural, socioeconomic, and healthcare contexts. The long-term use of technology, such as mobile apps and social media platforms, should be explored to support continuous education, motivation, and monitoring. Fourth, we developed the DPBS and tested it for validity and reliability. However, future studies are needed to further validate this tool to assess diabetes prevention behavior among individuals at risk for T2DM. Fifth, we used a quasi-experimental design to assess the effectiveness of a behavior modification model for T2DM in high-risk groups. This design is prone to internal validity threats like maturation, selection bias, and regression to the mean. The lack of random assignment makes it difficult to attribute observed effects solely to the intervention. Future research should utilize randomized controlled trials (RCTs) to overcome this limitation. Additionally, further studies will be necessary to explore the interactions between social media and evidence-based practice and to formulate institutional policies that benefit patients, clinicians, public health practitioners, and the industry as a whole.

5. Conclusions

Diabetes is a chronic non-communicable disease that leads to numerous complications. The current study aimed to develop a behavior modification intervention for preventing T2DM among individuals at risk and to compare diabetes prevention behaviors and fasting blood sugar levels between the intervention and comparison groups. Our findings revealed that the intervention group exhibited statistically significant higher average scores in nutrition, exercise, and stress management compared to the comparison group. Additionally, the intervention group demonstrated significantly lower average blood sugar levels. These results indicate that the behavior modification intervention had a positive impact on the food consumption behavior, exercise habits, and stress management of individuals at risk for diabetes. Additional research is needed to assess the impact of social media on the dissemination of knowledge in clinical practice and to determine whether it significantly enhances patient outcomes. Consequently, health professionals can leverage these findings to implement preventive measures against diabetes among at-risk groups, addressing this significant public health concern effectively.

Author Contributions: Conceptualization, T.P., S.T. and P.K.; methodology, T.P., S.T., P.K. and W.S.; formal analysis, T.P. and W.S.; investigation, S.T. and P.K.; data curation, T.P., S.T. and P.K.; writing—original draft preparation, T.P. and S.T.; writing—review and editing, T.P., S.T., P.K. and W.S.; supervision, S.T. and P.K. All authors have read and agreed to the published version of the manuscript.

Funding: This research received no external funding.

Institutional Review Board Statement: This study was conducted in accordance with the Declaration of Helsinki, and approved by the Institutional Review Board of Krirk University (protocol code 0201/003 and dated 1 October 2022).

Informed Consent Statement: Informed consent was obtained from all subjects involved in this study.

Data Availability Statement: The data sets aside from the research information of this study, are not publicly available due to information that could compromise the research participants' privacy. However, data may be shared upon request to the authors.

Acknowledgments: We extend our gratitude to the participants for providing valuable data. This study was partially funded for publication by Krirk University, Bangkok, Thailand.

Conflicts of Interest: The authors declare no conflicts of interest.

References

1. Sun, H.; Saeedi, P.; Karuranga, S.; Pinkepank, M.; Ogurtsova, K.; Duncan, B.B.; Stein, C.; Basit, A.; Chan, J.C.; Mbanya, J.C.; et al. IDF Diabetes Atlas: Global, regional and country-level diabetes prevalence estimates for 2021 and projections for 2045. *Diabetes Res. Clin. Pract.* **2022**, *183*, 109119. [CrossRef] [PubMed]
2. International Diabetes Federation. *IDF Diabetes Atlas*, 10th ed.; International Diabetes Federation: Brussels, Belgium, 2021.
3. Suksatan, W.; Prabsangob, K.; Choompunuch, B. Association between Health Literacy, Self-care Behavior, and Blood Sugar Level among Older Patients with Type 2 Diabetes in Rural Thai Communities. *Ann. Geriatr. Med. Res.* **2021**, *25*, 318–323. [CrossRef] [PubMed]
4. Cryer, P.E. Mechanisms of Hypoglycemia-Associated Autonomic Failure and Its Component Syndromes in Diabetes. *Diabetes* **2005**, *54*, 3592–3601. [CrossRef] [PubMed]
5. Aekplakorn, W.; Suriyawongpaisal, P.; Srithamrongsawadi, S.; Kaewkamjonchai, P. Assessing a national policy on strengthening chronic care in primary care settings of a middle-income country using patients' perspectives. *BMC Health Serv. Res.* **2021**, *21*, 223. [CrossRef] [PubMed]
6. Posai, V.; Suksatan, W.; Choompunuch, B.; Koontalay, A.; Ounprasertsuk, J.; Sadang, J.M. Assessment of the Health-Promoting Behaviors of Hospitalized Patients with Non-Communicable Diseases During the Second Wave of COVID-19. *J. Multidiscip. Healthc.* **2021**, *14*, 2185–2194. [CrossRef] [PubMed]
7. Beagley, J.; Guariguata, L.; Weil, C.; Motala, A.A. Global estimates of undiagnosed diabetes in adults. *Diabetes Res. Clin. Pract.* **2014**, *103*, 150–160. [CrossRef] [PubMed]
8. Valinsky, L.; Mishali, M.; Endevelt, R.; Preiss, R.; Dopelt, K.; Heymann, A.D. Reducing resistance to treatment, through group intervention, improves clinical measurements in patients with type 2 diabetes. *BMC Endocr. Disord.* **2013**, *13*, 61. [CrossRef] [PubMed]
9. Gupta, L.; Khandelwal, D.; Lal, P.R.; Gupta, Y.; Kalra, S.; Dutta, D. Factors Determining the Success of Therapeutic Lifestyle Interventions in Diabetes—Role of Partner and Family Support. *Eur. Endocrinol.* **2019**, *15*, 18–24. [CrossRef]
10. Asif, M. The prevention and control the type-2 diabetes by changing lifestyle and dietary pattern. *J. Educ. Health Promot.* **2014**, *3*, 1. [CrossRef]
11. Mukona, D.M.; Zvinavashe, M. Self- management of diabetes mellitus during the Covid-19 pandemic: Recommendations for a resource limited setting. *Diabetes Metab. Syndr. Clin. Res. Rev.* **2020**, *14*, 1575–1578. [CrossRef]
12. Thangthum, W.; Makkabphalanon, K.; Phawo, P.; Poolpol, W. The effect of the disease prevention enhancement program which applied protection motivation theory on disease prevention behaviors in people at risk of diabetes: Case study. *J. Roi Kaensarn Acad.* **2023**, *8*, 211–225.
13. TInkong, T.; Kurmud, W. Effects of self-regulation and group process program on eating behaviors, exercise and fasting blood sugar (FBS) of diabetes mellitus risk groups in Ban Lao Tama Sub-district Health Promoting Hospital. *J. Res. Health Innov. Dev.* **2023**, *4*, 150–163.
14. Jaranai, J.; Kraithaworn, P.; Piaseu, N. Effects of a family participation program by using the Ramamodelon health behaviors, nutritional status and blood sugar level in diabetic risk group in community. *Kuakarun J. Nurs.* **2016**, *23*, 41–59.
15. García-Molina, L.; Lewis-Mikhael, A.-M.; Riquelme-Gallego, B.; Cano-Ibáñez, N.; Oliveras-López, M.-J.; Bueno-Cavanillas, A. Improving type 2 diabetes mellitus glycaemic control through lifestyle modification implementing diet intervention: A systematic review and meta-analysis. *Eur. J. Nutr.* **2020**, *59*, 1313–1328. [CrossRef]

16. Sanaeinasab, H.; Saffari, M.; Yazdanparast, D.; Karimi Zarchi, A.; Al-Zaben, F.; Koenig, H.G.; Pakpour, A.H. Effects of a health education program to promote healthy lifestyle and glycemic control in patients with type 2 diabetes: A randomized controlled trial. *Prim. Care Diabetes* **2021**, *15*, 275–282. [CrossRef] [PubMed]
17. Idris, I.; Hampton, J.; Moncrieff, F.; Whitman, M. Effectiveness of a Digital Lifestyle Change Program in Obese and Type 2 Diabetes Populations: Service Evaluation of Real-World Data. *JMIR Diabetes* **2020**, *5*, e15189. [CrossRef] [PubMed]
18. Panpetch, S. The effect of a health behavior modification program on food consumption behavior, exercise, and waist circumference diabetes mellitus risk group in Niwet Tombol Health Promoting Hospital. *J. Res. Health Innov. Dev.* **2021**, *2*, 97–108.
19. Ratchaburi Provincial Public Health Office. Non-Communicable Diseases Dashboard. Available online: http://rbr.hdc.moph.go.th/hdc/reports/report (accessed on 15 May 2024).
20. Kanfer, F.H.; Hagerman, S. A Model of Self-Regulation. In *Motivation, Intention, and Volition*; Springer: Berlin/Heidelberg, Germany, 1987; pp. 293–307.
21. Ghahramani, A.; de Courten, M.; Prokofieva, M. The potential of social media in health promotion beyond creating awareness: An integrative review. *BMC Public Health* **2022**, *22*, 2402. [CrossRef] [PubMed]
22. Phithak, T.; Surasangprasert, P.; Kamollimsakul, S. Going beyond Chat: Designing Connotative Meaningful Line Stickers to Promote Road Safety in Thailand through Participatory Design. *Safety* **2023**, *9*, 87. [CrossRef]
23. Kang, H. Sample size determination and power analysis using the G*Power software. *J. Educ. Eval. Health Prof.* **2021**, *18*, 17. [CrossRef]
24. Antonijević, A.; Stojanović, E.; Jevtić, A.; Živković, V.; Bolevich, S.; Jakovljević, V. The effect of a 6-month walking program on biochemical parameters in sedentary adults with type 2 diabetes mellitus. *Nagoya J. Med. Sci.* **2022**, *84*, 580–592. [CrossRef] [PubMed]
25. Diabetes Association of Thailand. *Clinical Practice Guideline for Diabetes 2017*; Diabetes Association of Thailand: Bangkok, Thailand, 2017.
26. Tang, Y.; Hew, K.F.; Herring, S.C.; Chen, Q. (Mis)communication through stickers in online group discussions: A multiple-case study. *Discourse Commun.* **2021**, *15*, 582–606. [CrossRef]
27. Gamboa Moreno, E.; Ochoa de Retana Garcia, L.; Del Campo Pena, M.E.; Sánchez Perez, Á.; Martinez Carazo, C.; Arbonies Ortiz, J.C.; Rua Portu, M.A.; Piñera Elorriaga, K.; Zenarutzabeitia Pikatza, A.; Urquiza Bengoa, M.N.; et al. A Pilot Study to Assess the Feasibility of the Spanish Diabetes Self-Management Program in the Basque Country. *J. Diabetes Res.* **2016**, *2016*, 9145673. [CrossRef] [PubMed]
28. Spring, B.; Champion, K.E.; Acabchuk, R.; Hennessy, E.A. Self-regulatory behaviour change techniques in interventions to promote healthy eating, physical activity, or weight loss: A meta-review. *Health Psychol. Rev.* **2021**, *15*, 508–539. [CrossRef] [PubMed]
29. Mungtaweepongsa, S.; Rasameethong, R. The effect of empowering home visit using the family genogram for prevention of dia-betes mellitus and hypertension among high risk population. *J. Nurs. Ther. Care* **2019**, *37*, 148–156.
30. Wilson, T.E.; Hennessy, E.A.; Falzon, L.; Boyd, R.; Kronish, I.M.; Birk, J.L. Effectiveness of interventions targeting self-regulation to improve adherence to chronic disease medications: A meta-review of meta-analyses. *Health Psychol. Rev.* **2020**, *14*, 66–85. [CrossRef]
31. Suksatan, W.; Tankumpuan, T. Mind–Body Interventions in Patients With Heart Failure: State of the Science. *J. Appl. Gerontol.* **2021**, *41*, 1232–1243. [CrossRef]
32. Ong-Artborirak, P.; Seangpraw, K.; Boonyathee, S.; Auttama, N.; Winaiprasert, P. Health literacy, self-efficacy, self-care behaviors, and glycemic control among older adults with type 2 diabetes mellitus: A cross-sectional study in Thai communities. *BMC Geriatr.* **2023**, *23*, 297. [CrossRef]

European Journal of
Investigation in Health, Psychology and Education

MDPI

Article

Association Between the Information Environment, Knowledge, Perceived Lack of Information, and Uptake of the HPV Vaccine in Female and Male Undergraduate Students in Belgrade, Serbia

Stefan Mandić-Rajčević [1,2,*], Vida Jeremić Stojković [3], Mila Paunić [4], Snežana Stojanović Ristić [4], Marija Obradović [4], Dejana Vuković [1,2] and Smiljana Cvjetković [3]

1 Institute of Social Medicine, Faculty of Medicine, University of Belgrade, 11000 Belgrade, Serbia; dejana.vukovic@med.bg.ac.rs
2 School of Public Health and Health Management, Faculty of Medicine, University of Belgrade, 11000 Belgrade, Serbia
3 Department of Humanities, Faculty of Medicine, University of Belgrade, 11000 Belgrade, Serbia; vida.jeremic-stojkovic@med.bg.ac.rs (V.J.S.); smiljana.cvjetkovic@med.bg.ac.rs (S.C.)
4 Institute for Students' Health of Belgrade, 11000 Belgrade, Serbia; mila.paunic@zzzzsbg.rs (M.P.); opsta.medicina@zzzzsbg.rs (S.S.R.); ginekologija@zzzzsbg.rs (M.O.)
* Correspondence: stefan.mandic-rajcevic@med.bg.ac.rs

Abstract: The aim of this study was to assess the association between the use of and trust in sources of information, knowledge about human papillomavirus (HPV) and vaccines against it, perceived lack of information, and the decision to receive the HPV vaccine in undergraduate students in Belgrade. The sample of this cross-sectional study included students aged 18 to 27 who received the second dose of the HPV vaccine or used other services of the general medicine department at the Institute for Students' Health of Belgrade during the period June–July 2024. The research instrument was a questionnaire consisting of socio-demographic data, information environment (sources of information, trust in sources of information, as well as questions related to perceived lack of information), knowledge about HPV and HPV vaccines, and vaccination status. Participants filled out an online questionnaire created on the RedCap platform of the Faculty of Medicine, University of Belgrade, which they accessed via a QR code. Hierarchical logistic regression was used to assess the association between vaccine status and socio-demographic characteristics, use and trust in information sources, knowledge, and perceived lack of information. Of the 603 participants who filled out the questionnaire completely, 78.6% were vaccinated against HPV. Key factors associated with vaccine uptake were female gender (OR = 2.33, $p < 0.05$), use of scientific literature (OR = 1.40, $p < 0.05$) and family as a source of information (OR = 1.37, $p < 0.01$), less frequent use of regional TV channels (OR = 0.76, $p < 0.05$), higher level of knowledge (OR = 1.43, $p < 0.01$), and lower perceived lack of information (OR = 0.50, $p < 0.01$). These variables explained 41% of variability in vaccine uptake in the multivariate hierarchical logistic regression model. Exposure to and trust in sources of information were significantly associated with knowledge about HPV and HPV vaccination, as well as with the perceived lack of information regarding HPV vaccination, and were the most significant determinants of the decision to accept HPV vaccine in the student population.

Keywords: human papilloma viruses; vaccine uptake; health behavior; infodemic; information ecosystem

1. Introduction

With 660,000 new cases and around 350,000 deaths in 2022, cervical cancer represents the fourth most common cancer in women globally, with the highest incidence rates and mortality in low- and middle-income countries (Bruni et al., 2023). In Europe, around 60,000 new cervical cancer cases are diagnosed annually, and in women aged 15–44, cervical cancer has the third highest incidence rate and mortality rate of 14.4 per 100,000 and 2.97 per 100,000, respectively. Serbia has the third highest age-standardized incidence rate of cervical cancer cases attributable to HPV of 18.7 per 100,000 women, surpassed by only Montenegro and Romania (Bruni et al., 2023).

HPV infection with "high-risk" types of HPV is a major cause of cervical cancer, with persistent HPV infection being a necessary factor for invasive cervical cancer development and responsible for 73% of new cases (G. Clifford et al., 2006; G. M. Clifford et al., 2003). HPV infection is associated with almost all squamous cell carcinomas of the anus, as well as carcinomas of the vulva (15–48%), vagina (78%), penis (53%), oropharynx (13–60%), and the oral cavity, and HPV type 16 is the dominant type in these carcinomas (de Martel et al., 2020). High-risk types, such as HPV-16 and HPV-18, are responsible for around 71% of carcinomas of the cervix, while together with HPV-45, HPV-31, HPV-33, HPV-52, and HPV-58, they are responsible for 90% of all HPV-DNA-positive squamous cell carcinomas (de Sanjose et al., 2010; Serrano et al., 2015).

Vaccination against human papillomavirus (HPV) is crucial for the primary prevention of cervical cancer, especially in low- and middle-income countries, due to the high mortality and low access to secondary and tertiary prevention (World Health Organization [WHO], n.d.). All registered vaccines are effective against HPV-16 and HPV-18, while the nonavalent vaccine also protects from HPV-31, HPV-33, HPV-45, HPV-52, and HPV-58, as well as HPV-6 and HPV-11 which cause genital warts. In the population of previously unexposed persons, the vaccine was shown to be 80–100% effective, and, in a study of over a million females, the risk of developing cervical cancer was 88% (95% CI 66–100%) lower in the group which was vaccinated before the age of 17 than in the unvaccinated group (Lei et al., 2020; Organization Mondiale de la Santé & WHO, 2022).

HPV vaccination rates vary significantly between European countries, ranging from 4% in Bulgaria to 90% in Portugal (for 2018) (Bonanni et al., 2020). Increasing HPV vaccination coverage faces many challenges globally, in Europe, and in Serbia, including lack of awareness, knowledge, and understanding of HPV infection and vaccination, concerns about vaccine safety and efficacy, perception of low risk, lack of healthcare provider recommendations, and general mistrust (Marić et al., 2018; Markovic-Denic et al., 2021; Štrbac et al., 2023). Many studies have demonstrated the important association between knowledge and HPV vaccine uptake. You et al. demonstrated that enhanced awareness among female college students in China significantly improved vaccination rates (You et al., 2020). Similarly, Al-Naggar et al. reported a strong association between HPV knowledge and vaccine uptake among schoolgirls in Malaysia (Al-Naggar et al., 2012). Xu further highlighted that understanding the cancer prevention benefits of the HPV vaccine is critical in fostering positive vaccination attitudes and increasing uptake among adolescents and parents (Xu et al., 2024). A systematic review by Addisu et al. confirmed a significant association between good knowledge and higher vaccine uptake, emphasizing the importance of informed decision making (Addisu et al., 2023). This finding was supported by Jiboc, whose systematic review revealed that better knowledge about HPV significantly enhances vaccine uptake among European women and adolescents (Jiboc et al., 2024). In Serbia, having a female child and knowledge about HPV were independently associated with a positive attitude towards vaccination among parents of children aged

< 9 years (Marić et al., 2018). Unfortunately, Rančić et al. have shown that, 10 years from the first HPV shot being administered in Serbia, only one fifth of students knew about the existence of the HPV vaccine and only 14.2% knew about both HPV and the vaccine protecting against it (Rančić et al., 2020). Factors such as knowledge, beliefs, and socio-economic environment have been shown to influence vaccine uptake, and the information environment is one of key factors influencing all of them and has recently been called a (social) determinant of health (Graham et al., 2024; Morley et al., 2020).

The information environment is defined as "constituted by all informational processes, services, and entities, thus including informational agents as well as their properties, interactions, and mutual relations" (Sequoiah-Grayson & Floridi, 2022). "Agents" include both individuals and organizations, and they also shape and contribute to their information environment, acting alone or as a group, online or offline, as information sources (Röttger & Vedres, 2020). The information environment, sources of information, and trust in information play crucial roles in influencing vaccine behavior. Previous studies have found that greater trust in primary physicians, official sources of information, and governmental sources, such as the CDC, was positively associated with vaccine behavior, uptake, or intention to receive vaccines (Bassler et al., 2022; Juarez et al., 2022; Okada et al., 2023; Purvis et al., 2021).

The HPV vaccine is primarily recommended for girls (women), aged 9 to 19 years old, and in countries with low coverage it is beneficial to also include boys (men) in HPV vaccination (Organization Mondiale de la Santé & WHO, 2022). In March 2022 the Health Insurance Fund of Serbia (the Fund) made the nonavalent HPV vaccine freely available to young people 9 to 19 years old, while it is not freely available to undergraduate students or anyone above the age of 19. In April 2024, the Fund made a number of doses available to undergraduate students aged 19–26 through the Institute for Students' Health of Belgrade. During April 2024, almost 3000 students received their first shot of the nonavalent HPV vaccine and following the standard vaccine schedule (0, 2, 6 months) were to receive their second dose in June 2024. HPV vaccination provides benefits even to young adults aged 19–26, but studies on autonomous young adults who could also benefit from HPV vaccination are lacking, and factors influencing their decision could probably differ from those of parents (Cocchio et al., 2020; López et al., 2020).

The aim of this study was to evaluate the association between frequency of use of and trust in information sources, the perceived lack of information, and knowledge about HPV vaccines and the decision to get vaccinated against HPV in undergraduate students. We hypothesize that HPV vaccine uptake is associated with higher frequency of use of scientific and professional sources of HPV-related information, higher trust in that information, and higher knowledge. Also, we hypothesize that the lower perceived lack of information is associated with HPV vaccine uptake.

2. Material and Methods

2.1. Study Design and Setting

This was a cross-sectional study performed on a convenience sample of undergraduate students who use the services of the Institute for Students' Health of Belgrade (Policlinic). The Policlinic is a dedicated healthcare institution focused on providing comprehensive primary healthcare services to students of universities and vocational schools in Belgrade.

2.2. Study Participants

The study sample consisted of a homogenous population of undergraduate students in Belgrade (typical start of undergraduate studies at 18–19 years), representing the target group for HPV vaccination. All participants utilized the same primary healthcare institution for students in Belgrade. The key distinction within the sample is between those who opted to get vaccinated when it became available and those who did not, despite being aware of HPV and its vaccine. In June and July 2024, those who decided to get vaccinated in April accessed the general medicine department of the Policlinic to receive their second dose of the nonavalent HPV, while other students used the services of the Policlinic for other standard reasons (e.g., current infection, regular health check-ups, referral to another healthcare facility). The recruitment was performed by study team members and student volunteers with the aim to cover the morning shift and most of the afternoon shift at the Policlinic (from 8:00 a.m. to 4:00 p.m.) every working day. All students accessing healthcare services at the department of general medicine in the study period were verbally informed about the study and provided with printed information for study participants. If they accepted to participate, they were offered a QR code which linked to the Research Electronic Data Capture (REDCap) survey hosted on secure servers of the Faculty of Medicine, University of Belgrade (Harris et al., 2019) .

2.3. Ethical Approval

The study protocol was reviewed and approved by the Ethics Committee of the Faculty of Medicine (Decision No. 25/VI-6) and the Ethics Committee of the Institute for Students' Health of Belgrade (Decision No. 1321/2). Participants were informed about the study verbally, through printed materials, and through the electronic data collection system, and their consent to participate was a condition to continue with filling out the electronic data form.

2.4. Instruments

The instrument was constructed based on a literature review to include the relevant factors which compose the information environment of the study participants. It focused on information-seeking behavior (Díaz Crescitelli et al., 2020; Wilder-Smith & Qureshi, 2020), sources of information and trust in them (UNICEF, 2018), as well as knowledge (Patel et al., 2016), which could ultimately influence vaccination uptake.

The instrument included the following sections:

1. ***HPV vaccination status*** was measured by a single item assessing whether the participant took the HPV vaccine, with a binary (YES/NO) response;
2. ***Information sources' frequency of use*** was evaluated by twelve items inquiring about the frequency of use of selected sources of information regarding HPV vaccines, on a five-point Likert scale ranging from 1 "Never" to 5 "Regularly";
3. ***Trust in information sources*** was evaluated by twelve items inquiring about trust in selected sources of information, assessed on a five-point Likert scale ranging from 1 "Not at all trustworthy" to 5 "Completely trustworthy";
4. ***Perceived lack of information*** was evaluated with four items on a five-point Likert scale ranging from 1 "Strongly disagree" to 5 "Strongly agree", measuring difficulty to make a vaccination decision, confusion with information, contradictory information, and having all necessary information about the HPV vaccine. A higher score indicated a stronger feeling of a lack of information;
5. ***HPV-related knowledge*** was assessed with seven True/False questions about HPV and HPV vaccines with a "Not sure" option. The knowledge score was calculated by summing up the number of correct answers;
6. ***Socio-demographic characteristics*** included nine items: gender, age, place of birth, economic status, religiousness (scale, score from 1, indicating "Not religious at

all", to 100, indicating "Extremely religious"), study area, faculty, and marital/relationship status.

2.5. Pilot Testing

The instrument and the data collection system were tested in a group of students ($N = 20$) before the beginning of the study. The pilot testing was performed at the same place where the actual data collection would take place, using printed questionnaires which were filled out by the students coming to the Policlinic to receive their second HPV vaccine dose or for other reasons. The time needed to fill out the questionnaire was measured, as well as readability and understanding of all questions.

The questionnaire was estimated to take 10–15 min to fill out, which is the usual waiting time during the process of vaccination. The students found the questionnaire detailed, but understandable, with no questions representing an issue. Students also validated the list of information sources without suggestions to extend or reduce it.

During the pilot testing, a number of students (10%) had no awareness of HPV or HPV vaccines. This problem was seen in both male and female students. Considering the very specific topic and approach of the study, connected to the *decision* to get vaccinated, and the instrument, the study team decided to add a "pre-question" to the online survey which asked the participants if they are aware of the existence of HPV and HPV vaccines. In case they were completely unaware (answering "No"), the online system would block them from participating in the study and offer them the link to the webpage of the Ministry of Health and the Institute of Public Health providing information about HPV and HPV vaccination. This ensured that participants are those who were able to actually make the informed decision to get vaccinated (or not).

2.6. Statistical Analysis

The primary outcome (dependent variable) was HPV vaccination status (vaccinated vs. unvaccinated). The secondary outcomes were HPV-related knowledge and a perceived lack of information (continuous variables). Socio-demographic characteristics of the participants, frequency of use of information sources, trust in information sources, knowledge, and perceived lack of information were used as independent variables when the primary outcome was modeled.

Results are presented as count (%), means ± standard deviation, or median (25th–75th percentile) depending on data type and distribution of data. Groups are compared using parametric (t-test, ANOVA) and non-parametric (chi-square, Mann–Whitney U test, Kruskal–Wallis test) tests. Spearman's rank correlation was used to examine the associations between the sources of information and the trust in those sources. The value of Cronbach's alpha was calculated for the "perceived lack of information" scale which consisted of 4 items.

Linear regression was used to evaluate the association between the knowledge score and perceived lack of information (dependent variables) and socio-demographic variables, frequency of use of different sources of information about HPV vaccines, and trust thereof. The results of univariate and multivariate linear regression analysis are presented as the β coefficient and 95% confidence interval (95% CI).

Hierarchical multivariate logistic regression was performed to evaluate the association between vaccination status and independent variables. The hierarchical approach involves adding blocks of variables sequentially into the regression model to evaluate their incremental explanatory power. This allows for the assessment of how different groups of variables contribute to the prediction of the outcome variable—in this case, the likelihood of being vaccinated against HPV. Blocks were the socio-demographic characteristics of participants, frequency of use of sources of information, knowledge score, and perceived lack of information. Each group/block of variables was first used in univariate analysis, and variables identified as significantly associated with the outcome were entered into the hierarchical multivariate logistic regression. In this analysis, Nagelkerke R square was employed as a measure of the goodness-of-fit for the hierarchical multivariate regression models. Nagelkerke R square is an adjusted version of the Cox and Snell R square, designed to provide a more interpretable measure of explained variance for logistic regression models, ranging from 0 to 1 (Nagelkerke, 1991). The use of Nagelkerke R square in this context provides a clear and interpretable measure of how well each model fits the data, allowing for the comparison of the incremental contribution of each block of variables in explaining the likelihood of being vaccinated against HPV.

All p values less than 0.05 were considered significant. All data were analyzed using SPSS 20.0 (IBM Corp. Released 2011. IBM SPSS Statistics for Windows, Version 20.0. Armonk, NY, USA: IBM Corp.) and R 3.4.2 (R Core Team (2017). R: A language and environment for statistical computing. R Foundation for Statistical Computing, Vienna, Austria. URL https://www.R-project.org/).

3. Results

During the study period in June and July 2024, student volunteers estimated 1012 students used the services of the general medicine department at the Policlinic and were approached about participating in the study during their shifts. The online questionnaire was accessed by 877 students (86.6%), of which 5.2% ($N = 46$) had never heard of HPV or HPV vaccines, so they were excluded from the study and directed to the website of the Ministry of Health of Serbia and the National Institute of Public Health of Serbia website about HPV and HPV vaccines. Out of the remaining 831 students, 800 (79% of the estimated number of students who accessed the services of general medicine in the study period) accepted to participate in the study and filled out at least the socio-demographic part of the questionnaire. Six hundred and three students (75.3% of those accepting to participate in the study, 59.6% of those accessing the services in the Policlinic) completed the whole questionnaire and were included in the analysis. There were no statistically significant differences between the students who did or did not complete the whole questionnaire in gender, area of study, marital status, or income level, but students who did get vaccinated against HPV were more likely to complete the whole questionnaire ($p < 0.001$).

Table 1 shows students' socio-demographic characteristics by vaccination status. Unvaccinated individuals were more likely to be male (31.0% vs. 14.6%) and reported higher levels of religiosity (median 68.0 vs. 55.0). In terms of field of study, a higher proportion of unvaccinated participants were from natural sciences (15.5% vs. 8.6%), whereas more vaccinated participants are from medical sciences (31.9% vs. 22.5%). Unvaccinated individuals were more often in stable relationships (47.3% vs. 35.7%), while vaccinated individuals are more frequently single (59.1% vs. 44.2%).

Table 2 presents the distribution of frequency of use of vaccine information sources among students by vaccination status. The sources of HPV-related information that were mostly relied on in our sample were internet portals (used often and regularly by 49.4%), social networks (used often and regularly by 48.3%), friends (relied on often and regularly by 45.1%), family (relied on often and regularly by 38.%), and chosen doctor (relied on often and regularly by 39.1%). Vaccinated students were more likely than unvaccinated students to often and regularly use scientific literature (30.2% vs. 15.5%, $p < 0.001$), internet portals/websites (50.4% vs. 45.8%, $p < 0.003$), family (41.3% vs. 27.2%, $p = 0.021$), and often and regularly rely on friends (48.3% vs. 33.3%, $p = 0.005$) and their doctor (42.2% vs. 27.9%, $p = 0.009$) as the source of information about vaccines.

Table 1. Socio-demographic characteristics of study participants by vaccination status.

	All Participants N = 603	Unvaccinated N = 129	Vaccinated N = 474	p Value
Gender:				<0.001
Male	109 (18.1%)	40 (31.0%)	69 (14.6%)	
Female	494 (81.9%)	89 (69.0%)	405 (85.4%)	
Age (years)	22.0 (21.0–23.0)	22.0 (20.0–23.0)	22.0 (21.0–23.0)	0.012
Faculty group *:				0.047
Technology and engineering sciences	125 (20.7%)	29 (22.5%)	96 (20.3%)	
Sciences and mathematics	61 (10.1%)	20 (15.5%)	41 (8.6%)	
Medical sciences	180 (29.9%)	29 (22.5%)	151 (31.9%)	
Social sciences and humanities	237 (39.3%)	51 (39.5%)	186 (39.2%)	
Self-reported religiousness (1–100):	59.0 (22.0–76.0)	68.0 (50.0–82.8)	55.0 (16.0–74.0)	<0.001
Self-assessed financial status:				0.128
Very good	52 (8.6%)	19 (14.7%)	33 (7.0%)	
Good	225 (37.3%)	43 (33.3%)	182 (38.4%)	
Average	302 (50.1%)	64 (49.6%)	238 (50.2%)	
Bad	18 (3.0%)	3 (2.3%)	15 (3.2%)	
Very bad	2 (0.3%)	0 (0.0%)	2 (0.4%)	
I would rather not say	4 (0.7%)	0 (0.0%)	4 (0.8%)	
Relationship status:				0.004
Single	337 (55.9%)	57 (44.2%)	280 (59.1%)	
Married	3 (0.5%)	2 (1.6%)	1 (0.2%)	
In a long-term relationship	230 (38.1%)	61 (47.3%)	169 (35.7%)	
Other—It's complicated	18 (3.0%)	3 (2.3%)	15 (3.2%)	
I would rather not say	15 (2.5%)	6 (4.7%)	9 (1.9%)	

* Classification of faculties is based on the official organization of faculties at the University of Belgrade.

Table 2. Information sources about vaccines by vaccination status.

	All Participants	Unvaccinated	Vaccinated	p Value
	N = 603	N = 129	N = 474	
Scientific literature:				<0.001
Never	151 (25.0%)	56 (43.4%)	95 (20.0%)	
Rarely	110 (18.2%)	20 (15.5%)	90 (19.0%)	
Sometimes	179 (29.7%)	33 (25.6%)	146 (30.8%)	
Often	100 (16.6%)	12 (9.3%)	88 (18.6%)	
Regularly	63 (10.4%)	8 (6.2%)	55 (11.6%)	
National TV channels:				0.025
Never	209 (34.7%)	50 (38.8%)	159 (33.5%)	
Rarely	150 (24.9%)	21 (16.3%)	129 (27.2%)	
Sometimes	162 (26.9%)	33 (25.6%)	129 (27.2%)	
Often	61 (10.1%)	17 (13.2%)	44 (9.3%)	
Regularly	21 (3.5%)	8 (6.2%)	13 (2.7%)	
Regional TV channels:				0.003
Never	254 (42.1%)	54 (41.9%)	200 (42.2%)	
Rarely	145 (24.0%)	21 (16.3%)	124 (26.2%)	
Sometimes	142 (23.5%)	30 (23.3%)	112 (23.6%)	
Often	43 (7.1%)	15 (11.6%)	28 (5.9%)	
Regularly	19 (3.2%)	9 (7.0%)	10 (2.1%)	

Table 2. *Cont.*

	All Participants	Unvaccinated	Vaccinated	*p* Value
	N = 603	*N* = 129	*N* = 474	
Internet portals:				0.003
Never	61 (10.1%)	25 (19.4%)	36 (7.6%)	
Rarely	68 (11.3%)	13 (10.1%)	55 (11.6%)	
Sometimes	176 (29.2%)	32 (24.8%)	144 (30.4%)	
Often	192 (31.8%)	37 (28.7%)	155 (32.7%)	
Regularly	106 (17.6%)	22 (17.1%)	84 (17.7%)	
YouTube channels:				0.778
Never	212 (35.2%)	49 (38.0%)	163 (34.4%)	
Rarely	123 (20.4%)	23 (17.8%)	100 (21.1%)	
Sometimes	143 (23.7%)	32 (24.8%)	111 (23.4%)	
Often	93 (15.4%)	17 (13.2%)	76 (16.0%)	
Regularly	32 (5.3%)	8 (6.2%)	24 (5.1%)	
Social networks (Instagram, Facebook, Viber, Twitter, WhatsApp):				0.382
Never	76 (12.6%)	21 (16.3%)	55 (11.6%)	
Rarely	81 (13.4%)	20 (15.5%)	61 (12.9%)	
Sometimes	155 (25.7%)	33 (25.6%)	122 (25.7%)	
Often	170 (28.2%)	29 (22.5%)	141 (29.7%)	
Regularly	121 (20.1%)	26 (20.2%)	95 (20.0%)	
Family:				0.021
Never	107 (17.7%)	32 (24.8%)	75 (15.8%)	
Rarely	98 (16.3%)	24 (18.6%)	74 (15.6%)	
Sometimes	167 (27.7%)	38 (29.5%)	129 (27.2%)	
Often	147 (24.4%)	25 (19.4%)	122 (25.7%)	
Regularly	84 (13.9%)	10 (7.8%)	74 (15.6%)	
Friends:				0.005
Never	52 (8.6%)	20 (15.5%)	32 (6.8%)	
Rarely	86 (14.3%)	20 (15.5%)	66 (13.9%)	
Sometimes	193 (32.0%)	46 (35.7%)	147 (31.0%)	
Often	184 (30.5%)	28 (21.7%)	156 (32.9%)	
Regularly	88 (14.6%)	15 (11.6%)	73 (15.4%)	
Your chosen physician, or physician you visit most often:				0.009
Never	113 (18.7%)	34 (26.4%)	79 (16.7%)	
Rarely	87 (14.4%)	22 (17.1%)	65 (13.7%)	
Sometimes	167 (27.7%)	37 (28.7%)	130 (27.4%)	
Often	142 (23.5%)	17 (13.2%)	125 (26.4%)	
Regularly	94 (15.6%)	19 (14.7%)	75 (15.8%)	
Healthcare professionals in media:				0.606
Never	125 (20.7%)	33 (25.6%)	92 (19.4%)	
Rarely	119 (19.7%)	23 (17.8%)	96 (20.3%)	
Sometimes	186 (30.8%)	40 (31.0%)	146 (30.8%)	
Often	115 (19.1%)	22 (17.1%)	93 (19.6%)	
Regularly	58 (9.6%)	11 (8.5%)	47 (9.9%)	

Table 2. *Cont.*

		All Participants	Unvaccinated	Vaccinated	*p* Value
		N = 603	*N* = 129	*N* = 474	
Religious leaders:					0.020
	Never	498 (82.6%)	95 (73.6%)	403 (85.0%)	
	Rarely	48 (8.0%)	13 (10.1%)	35 (7.4%)	
	Sometimes	42 (7.0%)	16 (12.4%)	26 (5.5%)	
	Often	8 (1.3%)	3 (2.3%)	5 (1.1%)	
	Regularly	7 (1.2%)	2 (1.6%)	5 (1.1%)	
Government:					0.265
	Never	379 (62.9%)	73 (56.6%)	306 (64.6%)	
	Rarely	114 (18.9%)	25 (19.4%)	89 (18.8%)	
	Sometimes	85 (14.1%)	23 (17.8%)	62 (13.1%)	
	Often	17 (2.8%)	6 (4.7%)	11 (2.3%)	
	Regularly	8 (1.3%)	2 (1.6%)	6 (1.3%)	

Table 3 shows the trust in information sources by vaccination status. Scientific literature was perceived as the most credible source of information in the whole sample with 84.9% of surveyed students finding it very or completely trustworthy, followed by their chosen physician (75.8% assessed as very or completely trustworthy). More than half of responding students assessed family (56.5%) and friends (51.1%) as very or completely trustworthy sources of information. The least trusted information sources were the government (assessed as very or completely trustworthy by 6.4%) and religious leaders (assessed as very or completely trustworthy by 7.8%). Trust in scientific literature was significantly higher among vaccinated individuals, with 53.6% assessing it as completely trustworthy and 34.2% assessing it as very trustworthy, compared to 43.4% and 31.0% among the unvaccinated, respectively ($p = 0.002$). For primary physicians, 39.2% of vaccinated participants assessed their physician as completely trustworthy, and 39.0% as very trustworthy, in contrast to 35.7% and 31.0% of the unvaccinated group, respectively ($p = 0.009$). Trust in religious leaders differed significantly between vaccinated and unvaccinated participants, with only 3.8% of vaccinated participants assessing them as very trustworthy and 3.6% as completely trustworthy, while 6.2% and 3.1% of the unvaccinated express similar levels of trust ($p = 0.019$).

Table 4 shows the percentage of correct answers to questions (knowledge) about HPV and HPV vaccines by vaccination status. Vaccinated participants correctly identified that the HPV vaccine protects against oncogenic strains of the virus more frequently (90.9% vs. 57.4%, $p < 0.001$). A greater proportion of vaccinated individuals correctly understood that the vaccine is effective even if received after the first sexual encounter (80.6% vs. 46.5%, $p < 0.001$) and that it is not only for females (95.1% vs. 69.8%, $p < 0.001$). Vaccinated participants were also more aware that oncogenic strains of HPV can cause various cancers (91.4% vs. 68.2%, $p < 0.001$). While knowledge about HPV causing head and neck cancers showed no significant difference ($p = 0.196$), vaccinated individuals were more likely to correctly refute the statement that women diagnosed with HPV infection should not receive the vaccine (50.8% vs. 25.6%, $p < 0.001$) and that condom use completely prevents HPV transmission (48.3% vs. 27.1%, $p < 0.001$). Overall, the total knowledge score was higher among vaccinated participants (median score 5 vs. 3, $p < 0.001$).

Table 3. Trust in information sources about vaccines by vaccination status.

	All Participants	Unvaccinated	Vaccinated	*p* Value
	N = 603	*N* = 129	*N* = 474	
Scientific literature:				0.002
Not at all trustworthy	5 (0.8%)	3 (2.3%)	2 (0.4%)	
Slightly trustworthy	10 (1.7%)	5 (3.9%)	5 (1.1%)	
Moderately trustworthy	76 (12.6%)	25 (19.4%)	51 (10.8%)	
Very trustworthy	202 (33.5%)	40 (31.0%)	162 (34.2%)	
Completely trustworthy	310 (51.4%)	56 (43.4%)	254 (53.6%)	
National TV channels:				0.426
Not at all trustworthy	166 (27.5%)	44 (34.1%)	122 (25.7%)	
Slightly trustworthy	179 (29.7%)	35 (27.1%)	144 (30.4%)	
Moderately trustworthy	205 (34.0%)	41 (31.8%)	164 (34.6%)	
Very trustworthy	39 (6.5%)	6 (4.7%)	33 (7.0%)	
Completely trustworthy	14 (2.3%)	3 (2.3%)	11 (2.3%)	
Regional TV channels:				0.838
Not at all trustworthy	184 (30.5%)	45 (34.9%)	139 (29.3%)	
Slightly trustworthy	185 (30.7%)	38 (29.5%)	147 (31.0%)	
Moderately trustworthy	190 (31.5%)	38 (29.5%)	152 (32.1%)	
Very trustworthy	31 (5.1%)	6 (4.7%)	25 (5.3%)	
Completely trustworthy	13 (2.2%)	2 (1.6%)	11 (2.3%)	
Internet portals:				0.061
Not at all trustworthy	98 (16.3%)	32 (24.8%)	66 (13.9%)	
Slightly trustworthy	161 (26.7%)	32 (24.8%)	129 (27.2%)	
Moderately trustworthy	275 (45.6%)	50 (38.8%)	225 (47.5%)	
Very trustworthy	54 (9.0%)	12 (9.3%)	42 (8.9%)	
Completely trustworthy	15 (2.5%)	3 (2.3%)	12 (2.5%)	
YouTube channels:				0.297
Not at all trustworthy	139 (23.1%)	37 (28.7%)	102 (21.5%)	
Slightly trustworthy	176 (29.2%)	34 (26.4%)	142 (30.0%)	
Moderately trustworthy	239 (39.6%)	47 (36.4%)	192 (40.5%)	
Very trustworthy	38 (6.3%)	7 (5.4%)	31 (6.5%)	
Completely trustworthy	11 (1.8%)	4 (3.1%)	7 (1.5%)	
Social networks (Instagram, Facebook, Viber, Twitter, WhatsApp):				0.029
Not at all trustworthy	110 (18.2%)	36 (27.9%)	74 (15.6%)	
Slightly trustworthy	160 (26.5%)	33 (25.6%)	127 (26.8%)	
Moderately trustworthy	271 (44.9%)	47 (36.4%)	224 (47.3%)	
Very trustworthy	47 (7.8%)	10 (7.8%)	37 (7.8%)	
Completely trustworthy	15 (2.5%)	3 (2.3%)	12 (2.5%)	
Family:				0.738
Not at all trustworthy	25 (4.1%)	7 (5.4%)	18 (3.8%)	
Slightly trustworthy	52 (8.6%)	12 (9.3%)	40 (8.4%)	
Moderately trustworthy	185 (30.7%)	43 (33.3%)	142 (30.0%)	
Very trustworthy	199 (33.0%)	41 (31.8%)	158 (33.3%)	
Completely trustworthy	142 (23.5%)	26 (20.2%)	116 (24.5%)	
Friends:				0.276
Not at all trustworthy	18 (3.0%)	7 (5.4%)	11 (2.3%)	
Slightly trustworthy	37 (6.1%)	8 (6.2%)	29 (6.1%)	
Moderately trustworthy	246 (40.8%)	55 (42.6%)	191 (40.3%)	
Very trustworthy	218 (36.2%)	46 (35.7%)	172 (36.3%)	
Completely trustworthy	84 (13.9%)	13 (10.1%)	71 (15.0%)	

Table 3. *Cont.*

	All Participants	Unvaccinated	Vaccinated	*p* Value
	N = 603	*N* = 129	*N* = 474	
Your chosen physician, or physician you visit most often:				0.009
Not at all trustworthy	8 (1.3%)	5 (3.9%)	3 (0.6%)	
Slightly trustworthy	19 (3.2%)	7 (5.4%)	12 (2.5%)	
Moderately trustworthy	119 (19.7%)	31 (24.0%)	88 (18.6%)	
Very trustworthy	225 (37.3%)	40 (31.0%)	185 (39.0%)	
Completely trustworthy	232 (38.5%)	46 (35.7%)	186 (39.2%)	
Healthcare professionals in media:				0.003
Not at all trustworthy	56 (9.3%)	23 (17.8%)	33 (7.0%)	
Slightly trustworthy	108 (17.9%)	19 (14.7%)	89 (18.8%)	
Moderately trustworthy	221 (36.7%)	48 (37.2%)	173 (36.5%)	
Very trustworthy	131 (21.7%)	21 (16.3%)	110 (23.2%)	
Completely trustworthy	87 (14.4%)	18 (14.0%)	69 (14.6%)	
Religious leaders:				0.019
Not at all trustworthy	401 (66.5%)	72 (55.8%)	329 (69.4%)	
Slightly trustworthy	75 (12.4%)	18 (14.0%)	57 (12.0%)	
Moderately trustworthy	80 (13.3%)	27 (20.9%)	53 (11.2%)	
Very trustworthy	26 (4.3%)	8 (6.2%)	18 (3.8%)	
Completely trustworthy	21 (3.5%)	4 (3.1%)	17 (3.6%)	
Government:				0.633
Not at all trustworthy	340 (56.4%)	71 (55.0%)	269 (56.8%)	
Slightly trustworthy	109 (18.1%)	21 (16.3%)	88 (18.6%)	
Moderately trustworthy	115 (19.1%)	30 (23.3%)	85 (17.9%)	
Very trustworthy	22 (3.6%)	3 (2.3%)	19 (4.0%)	
Completely trustworthy	17 (2.8%)	4 (3.1%)	13 (2.7%)	

Frequency of use and trust in the respective information sources were moderately correlated (Spearman ρ between 0.5 and 0.6). After testing with both sources of information and trust in the sources of information, trust was excluded from the hierarchical multiple logistic regression analysis due to collinearity and providing no additional value to the model.

Table 4. Knowledge about HPV and HPV vaccine by vaccination status.

	All Participants	Unvaccinated	Vaccinated	*p* Value
	N = 603	*N* = 129	*N* = 474	
The HPV vaccine protects against oncogenic (cancer-causing) strains of the human papillomavirus.				<0.001
Correct *	505 (83.7%)	74 (57.4%)	431 (90.9%)	
Incorrect	12 (2.0%)	7 (5.4%)	5 (1.1%)	
Not sure	86 (14.3%)	48 (37.2%)	38 (8.0%)	
The HPV vaccine is only effective if it is received before the first sexual intercourse.				<0.001
Correct	33 (5.5%)	15 (11.6%)	18 (3.8%)	
Incorrect *	442 (73.3%)	60 (46.5%)	382 (80.6%)	
Not sure	128 (21.2%)	54 (41.9%)	74 (15.6%)	
The HPV vaccine is intended for females only.				<0.001
Correct	16 (2.7%)	10 (7.8%)	6 (1.3%)	
Incorrect *	541 (89.7%)	90 (69.8%)	451 (95.1%)	
Not sure	46 (7.6%)	29 (22.5%)	17 (3.6%)	

Table 4. Cont.

	All Participants	Unvaccinated	Vaccinated	p Value
	N = 603	N = 129	N = 474	
Oncogenic strains of human papillomavirus can cause cancer of the cervix, vagina, vulva, penis, anus, and oral cavity.				<0.001
Correct *	521 (86.4%)	88 (68.2%)	433 (91.4%)	
Incorrect	11 (1.8%)	7 (5.4%)	4 (0.8%)	
Not sure	71 (11.8%)	34 (26.4%)	37 (7.8%)	
HPV causes some cancers of the head and neck.				0.196
Correct *	174 (28.9%)	29 (22.5%)	145 (30.6%)	
Incorrect	96 (15.9%)	22 (17.1%)	74 (15.6%)	
Not sure	333 (55.2%)	78 (60.5%)	255 (53.8%)	
Females diagnosed with HPV infection should not receive the HPV vaccine.				<0.001
Correct	63 (10.4%)	17 (13.2%)	46 (9.7%)	
Incorrect *	274 (45.4%)	33 (25.6%)	241 (50.8%)	
Not sure	266 (44.1%)	79 (61.2%)	187 (39.5%)	
The use of condoms prevents the transmission of HPV.				<0.001
Correct	175 (29.0%)	39 (30.2%)	136 (28.7%)	
Incorrect *	264 (43.8%)	35 (27.1%)	229 (48.3%)	
Not sure	164 (27.2%)	55 (42.6%)	109 (23.0%)	
Total score (no. correct)	5.0 (0.0–7.0)	3.0 (0.0–7.0)	5.0 (0.0–7.0)	<0.001

* indicates the correct answer.

Table 5 shows items related to the perceived lack of information about HPV vaccines. Among vaccinated participants, 41.1% strongly disagreed with the statement that it is difficult to decide whether to get vaccinated due to insufficient information ($p < 0.001$), 43.2% strongly disagreed with being confused by incomplete information about the HPV vaccine ($p < 0.001$), 43.2% strongly disagreed with being confused by contradictory information ($p < 0.001$), and 40.1% mostly agreed and 33.5% completely agreed they had all the necessary information about the HPV vaccine ($p < 0.001$). The perceived lack of information as a scale included four items with Cronbach's α of 0.87. There was a statistically significant difference in the perceived lack of information between the vaccinated and unvaccinated individuals ($p < 0.001$).

Table 5. Perceived lack of information by vaccination status.

	All Participants	Unvaccinated	Vaccinated	p Value
	N = 603	N = 129	N = 474	
It is hard to make the decision whether to vaccinate against HPV, since there is a lack of information about vaccines.				<0.001
Strongly disagree	220 (36.5%)	25 (19.4%)	195 (41.1%)	
Disagree	138 (22.9%)	17 (13.2%)	121 (25.5%)	
Neither disagree nor agree	121 (20.1%)	38 (29.5%)	83 (17.5%)	
Agree	87 (14.4%)	27 (20.9%)	60 (12.7%)	
Strongly agree	37 (6.1%)	22 (17.1%)	15 (3.2%)	

Table 5. *Cont.*

	All Participants	Unvaccinated	Vaccinated	*p* Value
	N = 603	*N* = 129	*N* = 474	
Incomplete information regarding the HPV vaccines I come across make me confused.				<0.001
Strongly disagree	225 (37.3%)	20 (15.5%)	205 (43.2%)	
Disagree	146 (24.2%)	19 (14.7%)	127 (26.8%)	
Neither disagree nor agree	135 (22.4%)	48 (37.2%)	87 (18.4%)	
Agree	64 (10.6%)	26 (20.2%)	38 (8.0%)	
Strongly agree	33 (5.5%)	16 (12.4%)	17 (3.6%)	
Contradictory information regarding the HPV vaccines I come across make me confused.				<0.001
Strongly disagree	229 (38.0%)	24 (18.6%)	205 (43.2%)	
Disagree	142 (23.5%)	21 (16.3%)	121 (25.5%)	
Neither disagree nor agree	138 (22.9%)	47 (36.4%)	91 (19.2%)	
Agree	58 (9.6%)	21 (16.3%)	37 (7.8%)	
Strongly agree	36 (6.0%)	16 (12.4%)	20 (4.2%)	
I have all the information I need regarding HPV vaccination.				<0.001
Strongly disagree	34 (5.6%)	20 (15.5%)	14 (3.0%)	
Disagree	52 (8.6%)	21 (16.3%)	31 (6.5%)	
Neither disagree nor agree	121 (20.1%)	41 (31.8%)	80 (16.9%)	
Agree	216 (35.8%)	26 (20.2%)	190 (40.1%)	
Strongly agree	180 (29.9%)	21 (16.3%)	159 (33.5%)	
Perceived lack of information (scale)	2.0 (1.2–3.0)	3.0 (2.2–3.5)	2.0 (1.2–2.8)	<0.001

Supplementary Material S1 shows the univariate and multivariate logistic regressions exploring the associations between the knowledge score and perceived lack of information with the use of sources of information.

Table 6 shows the hierarchical multiple logistic regression analysis of variables significantly associated with vaccination status. The total score range for the continuous numerical variable "religiousness" was divided into quintiles for easier interpretation of the results: 0–20 (completely non-religious), 20.1–40 (moderately non-religious), 40.1–60 (neither non-religious nor religious), 60.1–80 (moderately religious), and 80.1–100 (extremely religious). Female gender (OR = 2.81, 95% CI: 1.59–4.95, $p < 0.01$) was significantly associated with higher odds of being vaccinated, while being more religious was associated with significantly lower odds of being vaccinated (OR = 0.22, 95% CI: 0.09–0.54, $p < 0.01$). The Nagelkerke R^2 for this model was 0.145, indicating a modest proportion of variance explained by only socio-demographic factors. In Model 2, the frequencies of using scientific literature (OR = 1.70, 95% CI: 1.35–2.13, $p < 0.01$) and family as information sources (OR = 1.46, 95% CI: 1.18–1.79, $p < 0.01$) were positively associated with vaccination, while frequent use of regional TV channels was negatively associated (OR = 0.71, 95% CI: 0.56–0.90, $p < 0.01$). The significance of gender persisted, and religousness remained a significant negative predictor. Information sources about HPV vaccines further improved the model's explanatory power (Nagelkerke R^2 = 0.255). Model 3 incorporated knowledge about HPV and vaccines, which increased the model's explanatory power (Nagelkerke R^2 = 0.355). Knowledge was strongly and positively associated with vaccination status (OR = 1.68, 95% CI: 1.41–2.00, $p < 0.01$), while the effect of using scientific literature remained significant but lower (OR = 1.33, 95% CI: 1.04–1.71, $p < 0.05$). Introducing perceived lack of information in Model 4 further improved the predictive power (Nagelkerke R^2 = 0.412). Perceived lack of information was negatively associated with being vaccinated

(OR = 0.50, 95% CI: 0.38–0.67, $p < 0.01$). The positive association with knowledge remained strong, and the information sources like scientific literature and family continued to be significant predictors of vaccinations status. Gender remained a significant factor, with females still more likely to be vaccinated than males (OR = 2.33, 95% CI: 1.18–4.62, $p < 0.05$). The final model, including socio-demographic variables, information sources, knowledge, and perceived lack of information, explained 41.2% of the variance in vaccination status.

Table 6. Hierarchical multiple logistic regression analysis of variables significantly associated with vaccination status.

Variable	Model 1 [a]	Model 2 [b]	Model 3 [c]	Model 4 [d]
	OR (95% CI)	OR (95% CI)	OR (95% CI)	OR (95% CI)
Gender				
Male	Ref.	Ref.	Ref.	Ref.
Female	2.81 (1.59–4.95) **	2.66 (1.42–4.99) **	2.02 (1.04–3.91) *	2.33 (1.18–4.62) *
Age	1.17 (1.03–1.32) *	1.17 (1.02–1.34) *	1.03 (0.89–1.19)	1.05 (0.90–1.22)
Religiousness				
Completely non-religious	Ref.	Ref.	Ref.	Ref.
Moderately non-religious	0.77 (0.26–2.31)	0.78 (0.25–2.46)	0.81 (0.25–2,64)	0.89 (0.26–3.02)
Neither non-religious nor religious	0.37 (0.15–0.94) *	0.40 (0.15–1.06)	0.48 (0.18–1.31)	0.52 (0.19–1.43)
Moderately religious	0.32 (0.13–0.77) *	0.37 (0.15–0.93) *	0.46 (0.18–1.20)	0.55 (0.21–1.47)
Extremely religious	0.22 (0.09–0.54) **	0.28 (0.11–0.75) *	0.31 (0.12–0.83) *	0.38 (0.14–1.06)
Faculty group *:				
Technology and engineering sciences	Ref.	Ref.	Ref.	
Sciences and mathematics	0.41 (0.17–0.95) *	0.40 (0.16–0.97) *	0.37 (0.14–0.93) *	0.34 (0.13–0.91) *
Medical sciences	1.41 (0.71–2.77)	0.90 (0.42–1.93)	0.84 (0.38–1.88)	0.60 (0.26–1.40)
Social sciences and humanities	0.81 (0.43–1.51)	0.77 (0.40–1.47)	0.91 (0.45–1.81)	0.92 (0.45–1.88)
Relationship status				
Single	Ref.	Ref.	Ref.	Ref.
Married	0.11 (0.01–1.45)	0.11 (0.01–1.62)	0.18 (0.01–2.27)	0.22 (0.02–2.87)
In a long-term relationship	0.56 (0.35–0.89) *	0.59 (0.36–0.96) *	0.60 (0.36–1.01)	0.48 (0.28–0.85) *
Other	1.24 (0.23–6.76)	1.45 (0.25–8.25)	3.20 (0.48–21.56)	3.34 (0.49–22.61)
Scientific literature (frequency of use)		1.70 (1.35–2.13) **	1.33 (1.04–1.71) *	1.40 (1.08–1.82) *
Regional channels (frequency of use)		0.71 (0.56–0.90) **	0.79 (0.62–1.01)	0.76 (0.59–0.99) *
Family (frequency of use)		1.46 (1.18–1.79) **	1.43 (1.15–1.78) *	1.37 (1.08–1.72) **
Religious leaders (frequency of use)		0.67 (0.48–0.94) *	0.90 (0.62–1.31)	0.89 (0.61–1.31)
Knowledge (score)			1.68 (1.41–2.00) **	1.43 (1.19–1.72) **
Perceived lack of information (score)				0.50 (0.38–0.67) **
Nagelkerke R^2	0.145	0.255	0.355	0.412

* $p < 0.05$; ** $p < 0.01$; [a] Model 1 includes socio-demographic variables; [b] Model 2 adds information sources about HPV vaccines; [c] Model 3 adds knowledge about HPV and vaccines; [d] Model 4 adds perceived lack of information.

4. Discussion

The present study underlines the important associations between the information environment, consisting of information agents acting as information sources and the trust in them, knowledge about HPV and HPV vaccines, and perceived lack of information, in the decision to get vaccinated against HPV in a population of male and female undergraduate students. HPV vaccine uptake was most strongly associated with the female gender, lower religiousness, use of and trust in scientific literature, national TV channels, internet portals, family, friends, and chosen doctor, low exposure and trust in religious leaders, higher knowledge about HPV and HPV vaccines, and lower perceived lack of information about HPV and HPV vaccines. To our knowledge this is among the first studies exploring the influence of information environment on HPV vaccine uptake among students as representatives of young adults.

Gender was strongly associated with vaccine uptake in our study, with 85% of vaccinated students being female. In a previous study conducted in southeast Serbia, girls had a four times higher vaccination rate than boys (Rančić et al., 2020). Similar results are seen in studies around the world where vaccination rates were 3–4 times higher in females than in males (Barnard et al., 2017). Vaccination of females has been a priority since the first registration of the vaccine, and previous studies have found that the HPV vaccine was in much later stages of adoption among females, with over 85% who had heard of HPV vaccines, compared with males, who have shown much lower knowledge and interest, underlining much higher media coverage prioritizing females (Kellogg et al., 2019; Kelly et al., 2009; Reiter et al., 2011; Wu et al., 2023). The pilot testing of our questionnaire had shown that a number of students might be completely unaware of HPV and the HPV vaccine, and in our study that number was 45 (5.2%) of the approached students, although it is possible that some of the students who refused to participate in the study were also unaware of HPV and HPV vaccines. In a sample of college students aged 18 years and older at California State University in Los Angeles County, more than half of male and female students did not know that the HPV vaccine is recommended for their age group (Kellogg et al., 2019), which indicates a relatively high awareness (~95%) of the students in Serbia.

Religiousness, often defined as the degree of religious commitment, affiliation, beliefs, and practices within a specific religious context, can play an important role in HPV vaccine uptake. A previous study aiming at filling the identified gap in understanding the relationship between religious commitment and HPV vaccination uptake, focusing on how strong religious commitment in young adults influences vaccination decisions, found that highly religious young adults had low knowledge of HPV and HPV vaccination, and religious beliefs were associated with lower HPV vaccination uptake (Birmingham et al., 2019). Since then, studies have found religiousness to have a negative, positive, or no association with HPV vaccine uptake (Grandahl et al., 2017; Shelton et al., 2013). In our study, religiousness, religious leaders as the source of information, and trust in religious leaders were negatively associated with knowledge about HPV, HPV vaccines, and vaccine uptake and positively associated with perceived lack of information. Nevertheless, in a recent study, Coleman et al. have indicated that single-item indices, also used in our study, although most common in the literature, may not be best suited to provide actionable insight regarding the religious beliefs/teachings which influence vaccine decisions (Coleman et al., 2024). Therefore, a more detailed, qualitative exploration of this association is warranted.

In our study, the most used information sources about HPV and HPV vaccines were internet portals, social networks, friends and family, and a chosen (personal) doctor, while the least used information sources were religious leaders and the government. Frequent reliance on the internet and family/friends was observed in a study of Hungarian high school seniors, where healthcare professionals played only a marginal role in providing information for this study sample, which was explained by less frequent contact with the healthcare system in this age group (Balla et al., 2016). Results similar to ours were obtained in a survey of college students in Beijing (China), where the primary sources of

HPV-related information were social media, college education, families or friends, and doctors or healthcare workers (Liu et al., 2020).

There was a moderate correlation between the frequency of use of specific information sources and the trust in those information sources. In fact, although surveyed students relied most frequently on information sources such as internet portals and social media, only 11.5%, and 10.2% trusted information obtained from internet portals and social media, respectively. On the other hand, scientific literature as the most trusted source is used often and regularly by less than one third of the students. UNICEF's "Changing Childhood Project" also revealed that young people rely on social media and internet portals but do not trust them, and the greatest trust in the accuracy of information was placed on that from healthcare workers, scientists, family, and friends (UNICEF, n.d.). This discrepancy can be explained by the fact that social media platforms are deeply ingrained in the daily lives of young people, and because they are so easily accessible, young people often rely on them out of habit or convenience, even if they have reservations about their credibility. Young people might rely on social media for quick updates but (should?) turn to more trusted sources (e.g., scientific literature, healthcare workers) for verifying important information, such as vaccine-related facts. Social media can significantly shape knowledge, attitudes, and behaviors on HPV vaccine uptake among undergraduate students. Social media platforms can enhance awareness and knowledge about HPV, as well as exposure to positive information that fosters favorable attitudes toward vaccination (Garg et al., 2024; Lama et al., 2021).

Our results show that students who were vaccinated against HPV relied on and trusted different sources of information compared to students who were not vaccinated. Using and trusting information from scientific literature, internet portals, and a chosen doctor were positively associated with higher knowledge about HPV and vaccine uptake and negatively associated with perceived lack of information to make a decision about HPV vaccination. On the other hand, using and trusting information from regional TV channels, the government, and religious leaders were negatively associated with knowledge and HPV vaccine uptake and positively associated with perceived lack of information. Vaccinated college students trusted the scientific literature, their chosen doctor, and healthcare workers from the media significantly more, while unvaccinated college students trusted religious leaders significantly more, although trust in most information sources was generally lower among unvaccinated individuals. Similar results were obtained in the study of drivers of HPV vaccine uptake among Italian university students, where students who relied on HPV-related information from healthcare workers and family members had higher inclination to get vaccinated (Cocchio et al., 2020), implying that healthcare and family settings can be very effective in driving health-related choices. Also, our findings that students who used scientific literature as a source of information more often manifested a higher level of HPV-related knowledge, felt better informed, and were more likely to get vaccinated highlight the importance of trusted, reliable sources in health education. Students who access and trust high-quality information are better equipped to make informed health decisions.

The majority of surveyed students knew that the HPV vaccine protects against oncogenic strains of human papilloma virus, that it can be received by both males and females, and that it can be effective even after the initiation of sexual activity. Regarding the diseases that can be prevented by vaccination, 86.4% new that the HPV causes cervical, vulvar, anal, penile, and oral cancer, and around one third knew that HPV can also cause some head and neck cancers. In a study of HPV-related knowledge of and attitudes towards HPV vaccination of Hungarian high school seniors, around two thirds knew that HPV can cause cervical cancer, while only small minority (below 10%) were aware of other pathologies caused by the virus in the anogenital region (Balla et al., 2016). Vaccinated students had higher HPV-related knowledge and felt better informed about the HPV vaccine compared to their unvaccinated counterparts. The level of HPV-related knowledge was positively associated with use of information coming from scientific literature and internet portals and negatively associated with the frequent use of national TV channels, religious leaders, and the government as information sources. Those students who more frequently relied on scientific literature felt more informed, unlike students who more frequently relied on religious leaders and YouTube channels who perceived a greater lack of information. Knowledge as a predictor of vaccination decisions was established previously (Díaz Crescitelli et al., 2020; Kalaij et al., 2021) and was confirmed as a predictor of HPV vaccination in several studies (Liu et al., 2020; Natipagon-Shah et al., 2021; Nuño et al., 2016), including our study.

The hierarchical multiple logistic regression analysis revealed how each additional block of variables changes the associations of previously introduced variables, while increasing the predictive power of the model. Gender and religiousness were significant predictors of vaccine uptake in the first model, but introducing information sources, such as scientific literature, regional channels, family, and religious leaders, in the second model reduced the strength of association between religiousness and vaccination uptake. In the final model, gender, scientific literature, regional channels, and family among information sources, knowledge, and perceived lack of information remained significant predictors of vaccination uptake.

Our results have demonstrated the strong relationship between the information environment, consisting of information sources and trust in them, and both knowledge and a perceived lack of information. The perceived lack of information consisted of items about difficulty in making the decision, having incomplete or contradictory information, or having all the necessary information to make the decision to get vaccinated. Those items reflect the core definition of the *infodemic*, as "An overabundance of information, some accurate and some not, that make it difficult for people to find trustworthy and reliable information in order to make a decision about their health" (Briand et al., 2023). Therefore, the "perceived lack of information" measured the effects of the infodemic well and was shown to be a significant predictor of the HPV vaccine uptake.

The main limitations of this study lay in its cross-sectional design and the representativeness of our sample. The cross-sectional design of this study prevents us from claiming causality in the identified strong associations between the information environment and HPV vaccine uptake, although the "exposure" to the information environment de facto happened before the decision to get vaccinated against HPV. Yet, a longitudinal design would provide a clearer picture of how knowledge and attitudes toward vaccination evolve over time. In our sample, the HPV vaccine uptake was 78.6%, which is extraordinarily high, and is much higher than the Serbian national average which is estimated to be below 4% and in reports from previous studies in Serbia where the HPV vaccine uptake was 2% (Marić et al., 2018). The estimated coverage in Serbia is similar to that of Turkey, with the coverage of less than 1% in girls, but much lower than that of other European countries such as Scotland (80%), Norway (73%), or Switzerland (72.6%) (Feiring et al., 2015; Kose et al., 2014; Sinka et al., 2014). The higher HPV vaccine coverage in our sample results from the fact that our study was organized during the period when students were scheduled to receive their second dose of the HPV vaccine in a short period of time, and in this period, they were the primary users of healthcare services in the Policlinic. This also explains the result that vaccinated students were significantly more likely to complete the whole questionnaire, as they might feel more responsible and even grateful that they were given the opportunity to get vaccinated against HPV for free during this period. Considering that the aim of the study was not to estimate HPV vaccine uptake but to explore the association between the information environment, knowledge, and perceived lack of information and HPV vaccine uptake, both the cross-sectional design and the present sample serve the purpose adequately. One important advantage of this sample rests on the fact that we can be fairly certain that the students' self-reported vaccination status is correct, as they were accessing the Policlinic to receive their second dose of the HPV vaccine, which is a clear advantage compared to online surveys or in-person settings with the general student population (where we would expect to have only 2–4% vaccinated individuals). However, recruiting participants from a healthcare setting may introduce bias, as these students might already have higher awareness of HPV and vaccination, so including a broader student population might contribute to better generalizability of the results.

Future studies should dive deeper into the gender differences in the information environment, trust, knowledge, and perceived lack of information to propose gender-specific strategies to increase HPV vaccination. Qualitative methods could help understand why certain information sources are trusted, providing insights to refine communication strategies, and could also shed light on religiousness and religious beliefs and their association with HPV vaccine uptake. Further investigation into specific knowledge gaps or misconceptions about HPV and its vaccine could guide more targeted educational interventions. Additionally, examining cultural and social factors influencing trust and conducting comparative analyses across regions or countries could uncover unique trends or universal patterns to enhance global health strategies.

Our results show the predictors of HPV vaccine uptake in settings where young people can take ownership of their health and make the medical decision about vaccination, which in Serbia and many other countries include young people from the age of 15 (McLendon et al., 2021). Methods with proven success include utilizing peer education, especially combining the peer-expert narrative (Hopfer, 2012), providing access to reliable information sources (websites, brochures), especially at vaccination sites or campuses (Krawczyk et al., 2012), leveraging social media to share reliable information and scientific literature about HPV and vaccination (Ferreira et al., 2022), and training healthcare providers to effectively communicate the importance of the HPV vaccine (Osaghae et al., 2022), with an emphasis on health communication strategies that focus on cancer prevention benefits of the HPV vaccine which resonate well with college students (Tatar et al., 2017).

5. Conclusions

The information environment and trust in information sources are significantly associated with knowledge about HPV and HPV vaccination, as well as with the perceived lack of information about HPV vaccination, a potential consequence of the infodemic. Together, they present the most significant determinants of making the decision to get vaccinated against HPV in the student population. Strategies to improve HPV vaccine uptake among adolescents and young adults should focus on using the school and college environment to promote high-quality sources of information and build trust, increase knowledge, and reduce the "perceived lack of information" caused by the infodemic.

Supplementary Materials: The following supporting information can be downloaded at: https://www.mdpi.com/article/10.3390/ejihpe15020021/s1, Table S1: Univariable and multivariable linear regression exploring the association between the knowledge score and use of sources of information about HPV vaccines. Table S2: Univariable and multivariable linear regression exploring the association between perceived lack of information and sources of information about HPV vaccines.

Author Contributions: Conceptualization, S.M.-R., V.J.S., D.V. and S.C.; data curation, S.M.-R. and S.C.; formal analysis, S.M.-R., V.J.S. and S.C.; investigation, S.M.-R., V.J.S., M.P., S.S.R., M.O. and S.C.; methodology, S.M.-R., V.J.S. and S.C.; resources, M.P., S.S.R. and M.O.; supervision, D.V.; validation, M.P., S.S.R., M.O. and D.V.; visualization, S.M.-R. and S.C.; writing—original draft, S.M.-R., V.J.S., D.V. and S.C.; writing—review and editing, S.M.-R., V.J.S., M.P., S.S.R., M.O., D.V. and S.C. All authors have read and agreed to the published version of the manuscript.

Funding: This research received no external funding.

Institutional Review Board Statement: The study protocol was reviewed and approved by the Ethics Committee of the Faculty of Medicine (Decision No. 25/VI-6) and the Ethics Committee of the Institute for Students' Health of Belgrade (Decision No. 1321/2). Participants were informed about the study verbally, through printed materials, and through the electronic data collection system, and their consent to participate was a condition to continue with filling out the electronic data form.

Informed Consent Statement: Informed consent was obtained from all subjects involved in the study.

Data Availability Statement: Data available upon reasonable request to the corresponding author.

Acknowledgments: We would like to acknowledge the kind support provided by Ivan Soldatović of the Institute of Medical Statistics and Informatics, Faculty of Medicine, University of Belgrade regarding the statistical analysis. We would also like to acknowledge the help and support provided by the nurses of the Institute for Students' Health of Belgrade (Policlinic) and student volunteers who helped with the data collection. Finally, we would like to acknowledge the management of the Institute for Students' Health of Belgrade for supporting this study and making it their mission to improve and protect the health of students.

Conflicts of Interest: The authors declare no conflicts of interest.

References

Addisu, D., Gebeyehu, N. A., & Belachew, Y. Y. (2023). Knowledge, attitude, and uptake of human papillomavirus vaccine among adolescent schoolgirls in Ethiopia: A systematic review and meta-analysis. *BMC Women's Health, 23*(1), 279. [CrossRef]

Al-Naggar, R. A., Bobryshev, Y. V., Al-Jashamy, K., & Al-Musli, M. (2012). Practice of HPV vaccine and associated factors among school girls in Melaka, Malaysia. *Asian Pacific Journal of Cancer Prevention, 13*(8), 3835–3840. [CrossRef] [PubMed]

Balla, B. C., Terebessy, A., Tóth, E., & Balázs, P. (2016). Young hungarian students' knowledge about HPV and their attitude toward HPV vaccination. *Vaccines, 5*(1), 1. [CrossRef] [PubMed]

Barnard, M., George, P., Perryman, M. L., & Wolff, L. A. (2017). Human papillomavirus (HPV) vaccine knowledge, attitudes, and uptake in college students: Implications from the Precaution Adoption Process Model. *PLoS ONE, 12*(8), e0182266. [CrossRef]

Bassler, J. R., Redden, D. T., Hall, A. G., Ford, E. T., Chrapah, S., & Erwin, P. C. (2022). COVID-19 vaccine knowledge, attitudes, and practices in Alabama: The case for primary health care providers. *Journal of Public Health Management and Practice, 28*(6), 631–638. [CrossRef] [PubMed]

Birmingham, W. C., Macintosh, J. L. B., Vaughn, A. A., & Graff, T. C. (2019). Strength of belief: Religious commitment, knowledge, and HPV vaccination adherence. *Psycho-Oncology, 28*(6), 1227–1233. [CrossRef] [PubMed]

Bonanni, P., Faivre, P., Lopalco, P. L., Joura, E. A., Bergroth, T., Varga, S., Gemayel, N., & Drury, R. (2020). The status of human papillomavirus vaccination recommendation, funding, and coverage in WHO Europe countries (2018–2019). *Expert Review of Vaccines, 19*(11), 1073–1083. [CrossRef] [PubMed]

Briand, S., Hess, S., Nguyen, T., & Purnat, T. D. (2023). Infodemic management in the twenty-first century. In *Managing infodemics in the 21st century: Addressing new public health challenges in the information ecosystem* (pp. 1–16). Springer International Publishing Cham.

Bruni, L., Albero, G., Serrano, B., Mena, M., Collado, J., Gómez, D., Muñoz, J., Bosch, F., & de Sanjosé, S. (2023). *Human papillomavirus and related diseases in the world.* Summary report 10 March 2023. ICO/IARC HPV Information Centre.

Clifford, G. M., Smith, J. S., Plummer, M., Muñoz, N., & Franceschi, S. (2003). Human papillomavirus types in invasive cervical cancer worldwide: A meta-analysis. *British Journal of Cancer, 88*(1), 63–73. [CrossRef] [PubMed]

Clifford, G., Franceschi, S., Diaz, M., Muñoz, N., & Villa, L. L. (2006). Chapter 3: HPV type-distribution in women with and without cervical neoplastic diseases. *Vaccine, 24*, S26–S34. [CrossRef] [PubMed]

Cocchio, S., Bertoncello, C., Baldovin, T., Fonzo, M., Bennici, S. E., Buja, A., Majori, S., & Baldo, V. (2020). Awareness of HPV and drivers of HPV vaccine uptake among university students: A quantitative, cross-sectional study. *Health & Social Care in the Community*, *28*(5), 1514–1524.

Coleman, D. C., Markham, C., Guilamo-Ramos, V., & Santa Maria, D. (2024). Relationship between religiosity and HPV vaccine initiation and intention in urban black and hispanic parents. *BMC Public Health*, *24*(1), 265. [CrossRef] [PubMed]

de Martel, C., Georges, D., Bray, F., Ferlay, J., & Clifford, G. M. (2020). Global burden of cancer attributable to infections in 2018: A worldwide incidence analysis. *The Lancet Global Health*, *8*(2), e180–e190. [CrossRef]

de Sanjose, S., Quint, W. G. V., Alemany, L., Geraets, D. T., Klaustermeier, J. E., Lloveras, B., Tous, S., Felix, A., Bravo, L. E., & Shin, H.-R. (2010). Human papillomavirus genotype attribution in invasive cervical cancer: A retrospective cross-sectional worldwide study. *The Lancet Oncology*, *11*(11), 1048–1056. [CrossRef] [PubMed]

Díaz Crescitelli, M. E., Ghirotto, L., Sisson, H., Sarli, L., Artioli, G., Bassi, M. C., Appicciutoli, G., & Hayter, M. (2020). A meta-synthesis study of the key elements involved in childhood vaccine hesitancy. *Public Health*, *180*, 38–45. [CrossRef] [PubMed]

Feiring, B., Laake, I., Molden, T., Cappelen, I., Håberg, S. E., Magnus, P., Steingrímsdóttir, Ó. A., Strand, B. H., Stålcrantz, J., & Trogstad, L. (2015). Do parental education and income matter? A nationwide register-based study on HPV vaccine uptake in the school-based immunisation programme in Norway. *BMJ Open*, *5*(5), e006422. [CrossRef]

Ferreira, G. R. O. N., Formigosa, J. A. da S., Lira, A. L. B. de C., Reis, R. K., Gir, E., Freitas, W. L. S., Carvalho, J. N., Gonçalves, L. H. T., Botelho, E. P., & Ramos, A. M. P. C. (2022). The family health strategy influence on the human papillomavirus vaccine acceptance in a peripheral community of the Brazilian Amazon region. *Health Equity*, *6*(1), 852–861. [CrossRef]

Garg, A., Nyitray, A. G., Roberts, J. R., Shungu, N., Ruggiero, K. J., Chandler, J., Damgacioglu, H., Zhu, Y., Brownstein, N. C., & Sterba, K. R. (2024). Consumption of health-related videos and human papillomavirus awareness: Cross-sectional analyses of a US national survey and YouTube from the urban-rural context. *Journal of Medical Internet Research*, *26*, e49749. [CrossRef] [PubMed]

Graham, G., Goren, N., Sounderajah, V., & DeSalvo, K. (2024). Information is a determinant of health. *Nature Medicine*, *30*(4), 927–928. [CrossRef]

Grandahl, M., Tydén, T., Westerling, R., Nevéus, T., Rosenblad, A., Hedin, E., & Oscarsson, M. (2017). To consent or decline HPV vaccination: A pilot study at the start of the national school-based vaccination program in Sweden. *Journal of School Health*, *87*(1), 62–70. [CrossRef]

Harris, P. A., Taylor, R., Minor, B. L., Elliott, V., Fernandez, M., O'Neal, L., McLeod, L., Delacqua, G., Delacqua, F., & Kirby, J. (2019). The REDCap consortium: Building an international community of software platform partners. *Journal of Biomedical Informatics*, *95*, 103208. [CrossRef] [PubMed]

Hopfer, S. (2012). Effects of a narrative HPV vaccination intervention aimed at reaching college women: A Randomized controlled trial. *Prevention Science*, *13*(2), 173–182. [CrossRef]

Jiboc, N., Paşca, A., Tăut, D., & Băban, A. (2024). Factors influencing human papillomavirus vaccination uptake in European women and adolescents: A systematic review and meta-analysis. *Psycho-Oncology*, *33*(1), e6242. [CrossRef] [PubMed]

Juarez, R., Phankitnirundorn, K., Okihiro, M., & Maunakea, A. K. (2022). Opposing role of trust as a modifier of COVID-19 vaccine uptake in an indigenous population. *Vaccines*, *10*(6), 968. [CrossRef]

Kalaij, A. G. I., Sugiyanto, M., & Ilham, A. F. (2021). Factors associated with vaccination compliance in Southeast Asian children: A systematic review. *Asia Pacific Journal of Public Health*, *33*(5), 479–488. [CrossRef]

Kellogg, C., Shu, J., Arroyo, A., Dinh, N. T., Wade, N., Sanchez, E., & Equils, O. (2019). A significant portion of college students are not aware of HPV disease and HPV vaccine recommendations. *Human Vaccines and Immunotherapeutics*, *15*(7–8), 1760–1766. [CrossRef]

Kelly, B. J., Leader, A. E., Mittermaier, D. J., Hornik, R. C., & Cappella, J. N. (2009). The HPV vaccine and the media: How has the topic been covered and what are the effects on knowledge about the virus and cervical cancer? *Patient Education and Counseling*, *77*(2), 308–313. [CrossRef] [PubMed]

Kose, D., Erkorkmaz, U., Cinar, N., & Altinkaynak, S. (2014). Mothers' knowledge and attitudes about HPV vaccination to prevent cervical cancers. *Asian Pacific Journal of Cancer Prevention*, *15*(17), 7263–7266. [CrossRef] [PubMed]

Krawczyk, A. L., Perez, S., Lau, E., Holcroft, C. A., Amsel, R., Knäuper, B., & Rosberger, Z. (2012). Human papillomavirus vaccination intentions and uptake in college women. *Health Psychology*, *31*(5), 685. [CrossRef] [PubMed]

Lama, Y., Quinn, S. C., Nan, X., & Cruz-Cano, R. (2021). Social media use and human papillomavirus awareness and knowledge among adults with children in the household: Examining the role of race, ethnicity, and gender. *Human Vaccines & Immunotherapeutics*, *17*(4), 1014–1024.

Lei, J., Ploner, A., Elfström, K. M., Wang, J., Roth, A., Fang, F., Sundström, K., Dillner, J., & Sparén, P. (2020). HPV vaccination and the risk of invasive cervical cancer. *New England Journal of Medicine*, *383*(14), 1340–1348. [CrossRef] [PubMed]

Liu, Y., Di, N., & Tao, X. (2020). Knowledge, practice and attitude towards HPV vaccination among college students in Beijing, China. *Human Vaccines and Immunotherapeutics*, *16*(1), 116–123. [CrossRef]

López, N., Garcés-Sánchez, M., Panizo, M. B., de la Cueva, I. S., Artés, M. T., Ramos, B., & Cotarelo, M. (2020). HPV knowledge and vaccine acceptance among European adolescents and their parents: A systematic literature review. *Public Health Reviews*, *41*, 1–24.

Marić, G., Birčanin, Đ., Kisić, V., Dotlić, J., Zarić, M., Kisić-Tepavčević, D., & Gazibara, T. (2018). Parental perspective on human papillomavirus (HPV) vaccination in Serbia: Knowledge, attitudes and practice. *Sexual and Reproductive Healthcare*, *16*(April), 192–198. [CrossRef] [PubMed]

Markovic-Denic, L., Milicevic, S., Todorovic, J., Nikolic, V., Djuric, O., Marusic, V., Dugalic, S., Vasiljevic, B., & Gojnic-Dugalic, M. (2021). Uptake of human papillomavirus vaccine and intention to vaccinate among healthy pregnant women in Serbia: A cross-sectional study on awareness, knowledge, and attitudes. *Viruses*, *13*(5), 727. [CrossRef]

McLendon, L., Puckett, J., Green, C., James, J., Head, K. J., Yun Lee, H., Young Pierce, J., Beasley, M., & Daniel, C. L. (2021). Factors associated with HPV vaccination initiation among United States college students. *Human Vaccines and Immunotherapeutics*, *17*(4), 1033–1043. [CrossRef]

Morley, J., Cowls, J., Taddeo, M., & Floridi, L. (2020). Public health in the information age: Recognizing the infosphere as a social determinant of health. *Journal of Medical Internet Research*, *22*(8), e19311. [CrossRef]

Nagelkerke, N. J. D. (1991). A note on a general definition of the coefficient of determination. *Biometrika*, *78*(3), 691–692. [CrossRef]

Natipagon-Shah, B., Lee, E., & Lee, S.-Y. (2021). Knowledge, beliefs, and practices among US college students concerning papillomavirus vaccination. *Journal of Community Health*, *46*(2), 380–388. [CrossRef] [PubMed]

Nuño, V. L., Gonzalez, M., Loredo, S. M., Nigon, B. M., & Garcia, F. (2016). A cross-sectional study of human papillomavirus vaccine utilization among university women: The role of ethnicity, race, and risk factors. *Journal of Lower Genital Tract Disease*, *20*(2), 131–134. [CrossRef]

Okada, H., Okuhara, T., Goto, E., & Kiuchi, T. (2023). Associations between Vaccination behavior and trust in information sources regarding COVID-19 vaccines under emergency approval in Japan: A cross-sectional study. *Vaccines*, *11*(2), 233. [CrossRef] [PubMed]

Organization Mondiale de la Santé & WHO. (2022). Human papillomavirus vaccines: WHO position paper (2022 update)–Vaccins contre les papillomavirus humains: Note de synthèse de l'OMS (mise à jour de 2022). *Weekly Epidemiological Record = Relevé Épidémiologique Hebdomadaire*, *97*(50), 645–672.

Osaghae, I., Chido-Amajuoyi, O. G., & Shete, S. (2022). Healthcare provider recommendations and observed changes in HPV vaccination acceptance during the COVID-19 pandemic. *Vaccines*, *10*(9), 1515. [CrossRef] [PubMed]

Patel, H., Jeve, Y. B., Sherman, S. M., & Moss, E. L. (2016). Knowledge of human papillomavirus and the human papillomavirus vaccine in European adolescents: A systematic review. *Sexually Transmitted Infections*, *92*(6), 474–479. [CrossRef]

Purvis, R. S., Hallgren, E., Moore, R. A., Willis, D. E., Hall, S., Gurel-Headley, M., & McElfish, P. A. (2021). Trusted sources of COVID-19 vaccine information among hesitant adopters in the United States. *Vaccines*, *9*(12), 1418. [CrossRef]

Rančić, N. K., Golubović, M. B., Ilić, M. V., Ignjatović, A. S., Živadinović, R. M., Đenić, S. N., Momčilović, S. D., Kocić, B. N., Milošević, Z. G., & Otašević, S. A. (2020). Knowledge about cervical cancer and awareness of human papillomavirus (HPV) and HPV vaccine among female students from Serbia. *Medicina*, *56*(8), 406. [CrossRef]

Reiter, P. L., McRee, A. L., Kadis, J. A., & Brewer, N. T. (2011). HPV vaccine and adolescent males. *Vaccine*, *29*(34), 5595–5602. [CrossRef]

Röttger, P., & Vedres, B. (2020). *The information environment and its effects on individuals and groups* (Vol. 30). Oxford Internet Institute.

Sequoiah-Grayson, S., & Floridi, L. (2022). Semantic conceptions of information. In *The stanford encyclopedia of philosophy* (Spring 2022 ed.). The Metaphysics Research Lab.

Serrano, B., de Sanjosé, S., Tous, S., Quiros, B., Muñoz, N., Bosch, X., & Alemany, L. (2015). Human papillomavirus genotype attribution for HPVs 6, 11, 16, 18, 31, 33, 45, 52 and 58 in female anogenital lesions. *European Journal of Cancer*, *51*(13), 1732–1741. [CrossRef] [PubMed]

Shelton, R. C., Snavely, A. C., de Jesus, M., Othus, M. D., & Allen, J. D. (2013). HPV Vaccine decision-making and acceptance: Does religion play a role? *Journal of Religion and Health*, *52*(4), 1120–1130. [CrossRef] [PubMed]

Sinka, K., Kavanagh, K., Gordon, R., Love, J., Potts, A., Donaghy, M., & Robertson, C. (2014). Achieving high and equitable coverage of adolescent HPV vaccine in Scotland. *Journal Epidemiol Community Health*, *68*(1), 57–63. [CrossRef] [PubMed]

Štrbac, M., Vuković, V., Pustahija, T., Nikolić, N., Rajčević, S., Ilić, S., Dugandžija, T., Patić, A., Ristić, M., & Petrović, V. (2023). Motives and attitudes of parents toward HPV vaccination: Results from the initial period of HPV vaccine rollout in Serbia. *PLoS ONE*, *18*(7), e0287295. [CrossRef]

Tatar, O., Perez, S., Naz, A., Shapiro, G. K., & Rosberger, Z. (2017). Psychosocial correlates of HPV vaccine acceptability in college males: A cross-sectional exploratory study. *Papillomavirus Research*, *4*(October), 99–107. [CrossRef]

UNICEF. (n.d.). *The changing childhood project*. UNICEF.

UNICEF. (2018). *Znanje, stavovi i prakse u vezi sa imunizacijom dece u Srbiji.* UNICEF.

Wilder-Smith, A. B., & Qureshi, K. (2020). Resurgence of measles in Europe: A systematic review on parental attitudes and beliefs of measles vaccine. *Journal of Epidemiology and Global Health, 10*(1), 46–58. [CrossRef] [PubMed]

World Health Organization [WHO]. (n.d.). *Cervical cancer: Key facts.* WHO.

Wu, H., Tong, X., Wang, L., Huang, Y., & Zhang, L. (2023). HPV vaccine information, knowledge, attitude, and recommendation intention among male college students in China. *Human Vaccines and Immunotherapeutics, 19*(2), 2228163. [CrossRef] [PubMed]

Xu, M. A., Choi, J., Capasso, A., & DiClemente, R. J. (2024). Improving HPV vaccination uptake among adolescents in low resource settings: Sociocultural and socioeconomic barriers and facilitators. *Adolescent Health, Medicine and Therapeutics, 15,* 73–82. [CrossRef] [PubMed]

You, D., Han, L., Li, L., Hu, J., D. Zimet, G., Alias, H., Danaee, M., Cai, L., Zeng, F., & Wong, L. P. (2020). Human papillomavirus (HPV) vaccine uptake and the willingness to receive the HPV vaccination among female college students in China: A multicenter study. *Vaccines, 8*(1), 31. [CrossRef] [PubMed]

European Journal of
Investigation in Health, Psychology and Education

MDPI

Article

The Impact of Pet Videos on Emotional Face Processing

Xingyu Zhu [1], Xiaojing Shi [2], Jiahao Liang [1], Bukuan Sun [2], Wuji Lin [1,*] and Jingyuan Lin [1,*]

1 Institute of Brain and Psychological Science, Sichuan Normal University, Chengdu 610066, China
2 School of Education, Fujian Polytechnic Normal University, Fuzhou 350300, China
* Correspondence: linwuji55555@sicnu.edu.cn (W.L.); linjingyuan921@sicnu.edu.cn (J.L.)

Abstract

In recent years, the number of people viewing pet videos and images online has risen. Although numerous studies have shown that owning pets positively impacts human mental health, the potential mental health benefits of prolonged exposure to pet media content remain debated. This study conducted three experiments to investigate how viewing pet videos affects human emotional face processing and to clarify the associated emotional regulatory mechanisms. Experiment 1 examined how viewing pet videos influences attentional bias toward emotional faces. Experiment 2 assessed the impact of watching pet videos on the valence perception of emotional faces. Experiment 3 analyzed how exposure to pet videos affects the valence perception of emotional text. The results showed that watching pet videos increased attentional bias toward subsequent positive emotional faces and decreased bias toward negative ones. This effect resulted from higher perceived valence ratings for both positive and neutral emotional faces. Importantly, this effect was only observed in facial stimuli with social attributes. These findings indicate that watching pet videos modulates emotional processing, and prolonged exposure to pet media content may affect mental health through this mechanism.

Keywords: pet video; emotion regulation; attention bias; emotion perception; emotional face

1. Introduction

The beneficial effects of pets on human physical and mental health have been substantiated by numerous studies (see review Wells, 2019; Liu et al., 2024). Pets are frequently recognized as vital sources of emotional support, with their presence demonstrating significant improvements in human emotional states (Janssens et al., 2021) and modulation of emotion-related neural activity along with alterations in neurotransmitter secretion (Liu et al., 2024, 2025). Cumulative evidence has established pets' therapeutic roles in stress reduction (Junça-Silva et al., 2022; Janssens et al., 2021; Rathish et al., 2022), anxiety alleviation (Kogan et al., 2021; Shearer et al., 2016; Hoagwood et al., 2022), depression mitigation (Brooks et al., 2018; Cheung & Kam, 2018; Hajek et al., 2024), and life satisfaction enhancement (Junça-Silva, 2022; Quan et al., 2023). Recent years have witnessed sustained growth in "pet-related" content across online video platforms. Humans demonstrate a higher preference for pet videos compared to most other video categories (X. Zhang et al., 2024; Si et al., 2025). Chronic indirect media exposure to pets appears to confer mental health benefits (S. Li et al., 2025), though the cognitive mechanisms remain underexplored due to limited empirical investigations. This study therefore employs three experiments to investigate how viewing pet videos affects emotional–cognitive processing, aiming to elucidate the cognitive mechanisms through which media-based pet exposure enhances mental health.

Multiple theoretical frameworks have been proposed to explain the mood-enhancing effects of pets. Bowlby's attachment theory posits that individuals form robust social bonds due to the security and support provided by specific entities (Bowlby, 2008). Recent research has expanded attachment theory to encompass non-human targets, such as pets, that can provide analogous feelings of security and support (Keefer et al., 2014). Attachment exhibits significant correlations with health outcomes, including emotional regulation, stress responses, perceived social support, and health-related behaviors (Taylor et al., 2024). Many pet owners identify pets as crucial sources of emotional support, with heightened attachment levels potentially mediating their psychological benefits (Langston, 2014). Additionally, the biophilia hypothesis proposes an innate human predisposition to affiliate with animals (Wilson, 1984). This inclination may confer adaptive advantages at the individual level (Mormann et al., 2011). The baby schema theory maintains that facial features like large eyes, small noses, and rounded contours elicit caregiving responses and positive affect in humans (Glocker et al., 2009). These positive emotional states evoked by pets contribute to enhanced psychological well-being. While these theoretical models collectively elucidate mechanisms underlying pets' mental health impacts, whether similar pathways mediate the effects of media-mediated indirect exposure remains unexplored.

Individuals respond to media content with reactions akin to real-life experiences (Mancuso et al., 2023; Z. Zhang et al., 2024). Lisa et al. (2004) demonstrated that participants exposed to the Cyberball task exclusion exhibited equivalent distress responses whether the exclusion originated from humans or computer agents. The content of media significantly affects the emotion experience of users when they use media and, in turn, influences their emotions and behaviors in real life (Z. Zhang et al., 2024). It suggests that media consumption of pet content may similarly impact psychological well-being.

Conversely, numerous studies have demonstrated that viewing pet videos and images alleviates stress and enhances positive affect (Ein et al., 2022, 2023; Na & Dong, 2023; Lavan et al., 2023). For instance, Ein et al. (2023) observed that participants who viewed pet videos prior to stress-inducing tasks exhibited attenuated stress responses during subsequent task performance. Lavan et al. (2023) reported significant increases in subjective well-being and physiological relaxation following three-minute exposures to puppy videos. These findings collectively indicate that indirect contact via visual media effectively modulates emotional states. This raises the critical question: Can sustained media exposure to pet content confer enduring mental health benefits?

Myrick (2015) assessed the mental health of individuals who watch cat videos and view cat images online through questionnaires. The results demonstrated that exposure to such content enhances positive emotions and reduces negative emotions, suggesting that media-based interaction with pets may benefit mental health. However, S. Li et al. (2025) compared the mental health of three groups: pet owners, non-owners, and people who frequently watch pet-related content online. The results found that pet owners exhibited significantly better mental health than non-owners. There was no significant difference in mental health between frequent online consumers of pet content and pet owners. While the frequent online consumers also showed no significant mental health advantage over non-owners. Moreover, the mechanisms by which pet ownership influences mental health differ from those linked to online exposure to pet content. S. Li et al. (2025) suggest that whether long-term media exposure to pet content can improve mental health remains to be explored.

While exposure to pet imagery and videos may enhance short-term emotional states, research on long-term outcomes remains inconclusive, and self-reported measures often fail to confirm causal relationships. Consequently, experimental research into the effects of pet media on human psychology holds critical scientific importance.

Aberrant emotional processing biases are prevalent in individuals with emotional disorders (W. Lin et al., 2021; Wei et al., 2024; Zhou & Shen, 2024). Targeted interventions

 https://doi.org/10.3390/ejihpe16020021

addressing these biases demonstrate efficacy in mitigating symptoms of emotional disorders (MacLeod & Clarke, 2015; Gao et al., 2022; J. Lin et al., 2024). If exposure to pet media influences cognitive–emotional biases, prolonged engagement with such content may alter mental health outcomes through persistent modifications in emotional processing.

Human faces exhibit high social salience and distinct neural processing pathways (Y. Li et al., 2024; J. Yang et al., 2024; M. Yang et al., 2024). For example, individuals tend to prioritize the processing of objects with social significance, such as faces (Y. Li et al., 2024). The mental health benefits of pets are mediated by their capacity to fulfill social support needs (S. Li et al., 2025). We hypothesize that pet media may modulate facial emotion processing through differential cognitive–emotional engagement. This study uses emotional facial stimuli to examine how exposure to pet videos alters emotion processing, thereby elucidating potential pathways linking media-based exposure to pets with mental health outcomes.

2. Experiment 1: The Impact of Pet Videos on Attentional Bias Towards Emotional Faces

Individuals with emotional disorders exhibit clinically distinct attentional processing patterns compared to healthy controls (MacLeod & Clarke, 2015). Building on evidence that pets elicit unique emotion-regulatory effects compared to nonsocial positive stimuli—potentially mediated by their social salience (S. Li et al., 2025)—this study rigorously compares how pet videos versus nonsocial positive stimuli (e.g., scenery videos) modulate attentional engagement with emotional faces, assessing both quantitative differences and qualitative mechanistic distinctions. The experimental paradigm investigates how exposure to three video categories (pet, scenery, and neutral) dynamically shapes attentional allocation to faces varying in emotional valence (positive, neutral, and negative).

Hypothesis 1 was that the attentional bias of the participants towards positive faces showed significant differences among the three conditions. The attentional bias in the pet condition was higher than that in the scenery condition, and the attentional bias in the scenery condition was higher than that in the neutral condition. Hypothesis 2 was that the attentional bias of the participants towards negative faces also showed significant differences among the three conditions. The attentional bias in the pet condition was lower than that in the scenery condition, and the attentional bias in the scenery condition was lower than that in the neutral condition.

2.1. Method

2.1.1. Participants

A medium effect size of f = 0.25 was used to conduct a power analysis with G*power 3.1. The estimated sample size needed was at least 34 participants to achieve 80% power and detect the effect given an α level of 0.05. The current experiment recruited 36 college students with normal or corrected-to-normal vision (23 females, aged 19.81 $\pm$ 1.49 years). None of these participants had participated in other experiments from this research.

2.1.2. Experimental Materials

(1) Videos

All stimuli were sourced from publicly available online repositories and standardized to 10 min silent clips. Pet stimuli exclusively depicted cats or dogs, excluding other species or human interaction. Scenery stimuli comprised natural landscapes devoid of fauna, humans, or anthropogenic elements. Neutral control stimuli consisted of digitally simulated film scratches, with white letters K and L presented centrally for 5 s at the 4 min and 8 min marks. A pilot study was conducted prior to the main experiment, in which 30 participants evaluated the emotional valence of 3 videos on a 7-point scale, with 7 being the most positive. Pilot experiment

https://doi.org/10.3390/ejihpe16020021

participants did not take part in any formal experiment. The purpose of the pilot study was to demonstrate that there is no significant difference in valence between pet videos and scenery videos, and that the valence of both is higher than that of neutral videos. A repeated-measures ANOVA with 3 (video type: pet, scenery and neutral) factors revealed that the main effect of valence was significant [$F(2, 58) = 102.304$, $p < 0.001$]. A post hoc test revealed that there was no significant difference between pet and scenery [$p = 0.702$], the pet was higher than the neutral [$p < 0.001$], and the scenery was significantly higher than the neutral [$p < 0.001$].

All animals shown in the videos met established indicators of positive animal welfare (e.g., expression of natural behaviors and positive mental states), following the consensus framework proposed by Rault et al. (2025), to ensure compliance with ethical research standards.

(2) Faces

Twenty-four negative, 24 positive, and 48 neutral facial stimuli were sourced from the Chinese Facial Affective Picture System (CFAPS; Y. Wang & Luo, 2005), with equal gender distribution (male/female). Each trial paired one emotional face (negative/positive) with a neutral face, forming 24 negative-neutral and 24 positive-neutral dyads. Neutral faces were counterbalanced across left/right positions within pairs to control for spatial bias. Trial types (consistent/inconsistent valence-side congruence) were equally distributed. Facial stimuli measured 7 cm (width) × 8 cm (height) on the display. The center-to-center distance between paired stimuli was fixed at 4 cm.

2.1.3. Experimental Procedure

The experimental procedure was programmed using Presentation 0.71 software. The participants sat in a seat in a soundproof room to complete the experiment. The background of the monitor was black, and the monitor was placed 80 cm away from the participant.

Participants completed three experimental sessions spaced at least three days apart. Identical procedures were followed across all sessions, with participants viewing distinct video categories in each session. A Latin square design was implemented to counterbalance video presentation order across participants.

Participants first completed a dot-probe task. Each trial comprised (1) a central fixation cross (+) for 500 ms; (2) a face pair displayed for 500 ms; (3) a 50 ms blank screen; (4) a probe (*) appearing for 2000 ms at one face location. Participants responded via keypress (F = left, J = right) to indicate probe position. Trials were classified as valence-congruent (probe replaced emotional face) or valence-incongruent (probe replaced neutral face). Congruent/incongruent trials and left/right probe positions were counterbalanced across conditions. (5) a 1000 ms inter-trial interval before the next trial.

After completing the dot-probe task, participants viewed a video, subsequently evaluated its valence using a 7-point scale, and responded to two attention-check questions. Any incorrect answer led to experiment termination and data exclusion (in fact, no participant was excluded). For the pet animal condition, questions included "Was a border collie present in the video?" and "Was a Garfield-cat depicted in the video?" Scenery condition queries were "Did the video showcase a starry sky?" and "Was a snowy landscape featured in the video?" Neutral condition questions asked, "Was the letter K present in the video?" and "Was the letter G displayed in the video?".

Finally, participants performed the dot-probe task again, with the same materials and procedure as the first task.

2.1.4. Data Analysis

Analyses were performed using SPSS 26.0. A measure of attention bias index was computed based on the work of MacLeod and Mathews (1988): Attention Bias Index (ABI) = $RT_{incon} - RT_{con}$. Specifically, the attentional bias index was calculated by subtract-

 https://doi.org/10.3390/ejihpe16020021

ing reaction times in congruent trials from reaction times in incongruent trials. A positive attentional bias index indicates that reaction times in incongruent trials were longer than those in congruent trials, suggesting faster responses in congruent trials and thus the presence of an attentional bias toward emotional stimuli. In this case, participants responded more rapidly to probes appearing at the location of emotional stimuli, whereas probes presented at the location of neutral stimuli required longer reaction times due to attentional reorienting. An attentional bias index of zero indicates no difference in reaction times between congruent and incongruent trials, reflecting the absence of attentional bias. A negative attentional bias index indicates shorter reaction times in incongruent trials than in congruent trials, suggesting faster responses in incongruent trials and reflecting attentional avoidance of emotional stimuli. In this case, participants responded more rapidly to probes appearing at the location of neutral stimuli and more slowly to probes appearing at the location of emotional stimuli, indicating avoidance of emotional information.

This study analyzed the difference between pre- and post-test attentional bias indexes as the dependent variable. Attention Bias Index Difference = ABIpre − ABIpost. The change in attentional bias was computed as the attentional bias index before video viewing minus the attentional bias index after video viewing. The more positive value indicated less post-video bias towards emotional stimuli. The attentional bias index (difference value) and video emotion valence were analyzed using a repeated-measures ANOVA, with post hoc comparisons conducted using the LSD test and the Bonferroni correction applied to adjust for multiple comparisons.

2.2. Results

A repeated-measures ANOVA on the attention bias index with emotion face (positive, negative) and video type (pet, scenery and neutral) as within-subject variables revealed a significant interaction effect between emotion face and video type [$F(2, 70) = 5.947$, $p < 0.01$, $\eta p^2 = 0.145$]. Simple effects analyses revealed pets were significantly higher than neutral [$p < 0.01$] in the negative condition. There was no significant difference between scenery and neutral [$p = 0.347$]. The difference between pet and scenery was also not significant [$p = 0.113$]. In the positive condition, pets were significantly lower than neutral [$p < 0.01$]. There was no significant difference between scenery and neutral [$p = 0.324$]. The difference between pets and scenery was also not significant [$p = 0.160$]. None of the main effects were significant (Figure 1 and Table 1).

A repeated-measures ANOVA on emotion valence of video with emotion valence (pet, scenery and neutral) as within-subject variables revealed a significant main effect [$F(2, 70) = 99.588$, $p < 0.001$, $\eta p^2 = 0.740$]. Post hoc tests showed that neutral was significantly lower than that for pet [$p < 0.001$] and scenery [$p < 0.001$]. There was no significant difference between pet and scenery [$p = 0.474$].

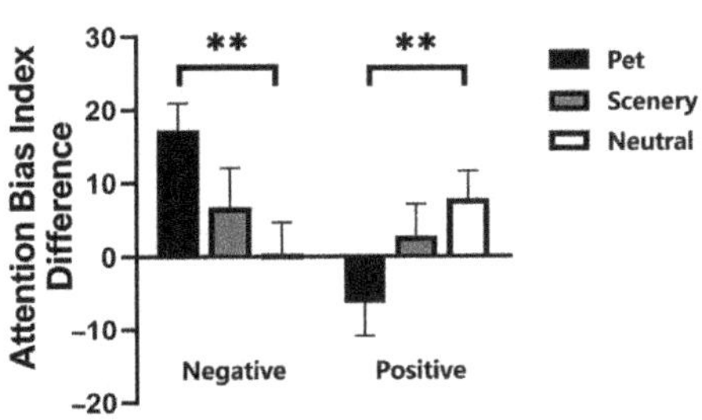

Figure 1. Attention bias index difference. Attention bias index difference = ABIpre − ABIpost. The attentional bias index difference was defined as the attentional bias index before minus after video viewing, with more positive values indicating reduced attentional bias toward emotional stimuli. ** $p < 0.01$. Error bars represent means ± SEM.

https://doi.org/10.3390/ejihpe16020021

Table 1. Reaction times and attention bias indices in the dot-probe task for each video condition and face valence. Standard deviation is presented in brackets.

	Face Valence	Pre-Video Viewing (ms)		Post-Video Viewing (ms)		Attention Bias Index (ABI) (ms)		Attention Bias Index Difference (ms)
		RTincon	RTcon	RTincon	RTcon	ABIpre	ABIpost	ABIpre-ABIpost
Pet	Negative	372.26 (86.33)	354.55 (86.17)	319.98 (67.69)	319.48 (63.99)	17.71 (31.48)	0.50 (41.72)	17.20 (22.30)
	Positive	352.75 (83.91)	344.70 (77.20)	342.01 (95.61)	327.58 (74.25)	8.05 (41.00)	14.43 (49.30)	−6.38 (27.41)
Scenery	Negative	377.11 (90.03)	360.89 (93.48)	328.80 (70.19)	319.21 (52.69)	16.23 (33.31)	9.59 (47.72)	6.64 (32.27)
	Positive	358.65 (82.18)	349.48 (72.04)	325.47 (66.21)	319.02 (49.27)	9.12 (22.87)	6.46 (34.71)	2.71 (26.33)
Neutral	Negative	422.62 (157.86)	408.59 (154.47)	374.12 (118.96)	360.47 (115.10)	14.03 (38.92)	13.65 (50.89)	0.38 (25.64)
	Positive	407.49 (161.39)	402.07 (164.53)	356.67 (109.94)	359.03 (107.94)	5.42 (30.00)	−2.36 (38.42)	7.78 (22.64)

2.3. Discussion

This study investigated how viewing pet videos influences subsequent emotional attentional bias. Findings revealed that after watching pet videos, participants exhibited a significant reduction in attentional bias towards negative emotional faces and a notable increase towards positive ones. In contrast, scenery videos showed no such effects.

Posner and Petersen (1990) divide the human attention system into several subsystems, two of which are relevant in the present context: orienting toward stimuli and disengaging from stimuli. The attenuated attentional bias toward negative-valenced facial stimuli suggests that pet-related video exposure decreases attentional maintenance on negative faces (greater orientation toward neutral faces) or facilitates disengagement from such stimuli (easier to disengage attention from negative faces) or the coexistence of both effects. Conversely, the heightened bias toward positive-affective cues reflects a reversal in cognitive prioritization patterns.

In the negative face condition, the attention bias index of the pet condition was significantly higher than that of the neutral condition. This result indicates that after the participants watched the pet videos, the time they spent looking at the negative faces significantly decreased. Watching pet videos can reduce people's attention bias towards negative faces. In the positive face condition, the attention bias index of the pet condition was significantly lower than that of the neutral condition. This result also shows that watching pet videos can increase people's attention bias towards positive faces.

While both the pilot and formal experiments demonstrated that pet and scenery videos had significantly higher valence than neutral videos, with no significant difference between them, their effects on attentional bias towards emotional faces differed. The pet videos used in the present study featured cats and dogs, which are the animals most commonly kept as companion animals in daily life. Unlike scenery videos, cats and dogs share close emotional bonds with humans. Liu et al. (2025) reported that viewing images of companion animals (cats and dogs) specifically activates brain regions associated with human attachment, as well as neural circuits involved in memory, emotion, and attachment-related cognitive processing. These findings suggest that viewing images of companion animals engages the human socio-emotional system. Furthermore, previous research has demonstrated that humans can form attachment relationships with pets, which provide emotional support and comfort (Keefer et al., 2014).

Therefore, we propose that the attentional bias–modulating effect of pet videos may not be solely attributable to positive mood induction but could also be related to the social support they provide. The social support from pets in videos may influence participants, altering their attentional bias towards socially attributed emotional faces. Conversely,

https://doi.org/10.3390/ejihpe16020021

scenery videos, although also inducing positive emotions, lack this effect. This indicates that pet videos exert a distinctive influence on human emotion regulation.

3. Experiment 2: The Impact of Pet Videos on the Valence Assessment of Emotional Faces

Experiment 1 demonstrates that viewing pet videos induces a specific alteration in participants' attentional bias towards emotional faces, yet the underlying mechanism remains unclear. A potential explanation could be a shift in participants' perception of facial emotion valence. However, if this attentional bias change is indeed attributable to altered emotional valence perception, when neutral and emotional stimuli are concurrently presented in experiments, it becomes impossible to discern whether the attentional bias change results from altered perception of emotion in neutral faces or emotional faces. Consequently, Experiment 2 aims to directly examine whether participants' subjective perception of emotional face valence changes following exposure to three video types, thereby further investigating the impact of pet information on emotional cognitive processing.

Hypothesis 3 was that the valence of faces in the pet condition was higher than that in the scenery condition, and the valence of faces in the scenery condition was higher than that in the neutral condition.

3.1. Method

3.1.1. Participants

A medium effect size of f = 0.25 was used to conduct a power analysis with G*power 3.1. The estimated sample size needed was at least 34 participants to achieve 80% power and detect the effect given an α level of 0.05. The current experiment recruited 36 college students with normal or corrected-to-normal vision (25 females, aged 20.94 $\pm$ 1.19 years). None of these participants had participated in other experiments from this research.

3.1.2. Experimental Materials

(1) Videos

Same as Experiment 1.

(2) Faces

Thirty-two negative, 32 neutral, and 32 positive faces were selected from the Chinese Facial Affective Picture System (CFAPS). There were equal numbers of male and female faces. Face pictures were presented at the center of the screen with a size of 7 cm by 8 cm.

3.1.3. Experimental Procedure

The experiment was conducted in the same sound-attenuated laboratory. Participants completed the experiment in three separate sessions, each spaced at least three days apart, during which they viewed three categories of videos (pet, scenery, and neutral) and completed the corresponding valence evaluation tasks. The order of video categories was counterbalanced across participants using a Latin square design to control for order effects.

At the beginning of each session, participants were seated 80 cm from the display monitor. The experimental procedure was programmed and presented using Presentation 0.71 software on a monitor with a refresh rate of 60 Hz.

Each experimental session consisted of three phases. First, participants watched a 10 min silent video corresponding to the assigned condition. Immediately afterward, they completed an emotional face valence evaluation task. In each trial, a white fixation cross was presented at the center of the screen for 500 ms, followed by the presentation of an emotional face (positive, negative, or neutral), which remained on the screen until a response was made. Participants were instructed to rate the valence of the face using

https://doi.org/10.3390/ejihpe16020021

numeric keys on the keyboard (1–7; 1 = "most negative", 7 = "most positive"). Upon response, the stimulus disappeared, followed by a randomly jittered blank interval of 1100–1500 ms before the next trial. The task comprised 96 trials presented in random order, including 32 positive, 32 negative, and 32 neutral faces.

Finally, participants answered two attention-check questions related to the viewed video and rated the valence of the video itself using a 7-point scale (1 = very negative, 7 = very positive).

The experimental environment, apparatus, video materials, and attention-check procedures were identical to those used in Experiment 1. The primary difference was that the dot-probe task employed in Experiment 1 was replaced by the valence evaluation task in the present experiment.

3.1.4. Data Analysis

Analyses were performed using SPSS 26.0. The emotional valence of facial stimuli and videos was analyzed using a repeated-measures ANOVA, with post hoc comparisons conducted using the LSD test and Bonferroni correction applied to adjust for multiple comparisons.

3.2. Results

A repeated-measures ANOVA on emotion valence with emotion face (positive, negative, neutral) and video type (pet, scenery and neutral) as within-subject variables revealed a significant main effect of emotion face [$F(2, 70) = 2644.913$, $p < 0.001$, $\eta p^2 = 0.987$] and video type [$F(2, 70) = 33.667$, $p < 0.001$, $\eta p^2 = 0.490$]. The interaction between emotion face and video type was significant [$F(4, 140) = 11.809$, $p < 0.001$, $\eta p^2 = 0.252$]. Simple effects analyses revealed neutral were significantly lower than pet [$p < 0.001$] and scenery [$p < 0.001$] in the positive condition. In the negative condition, there was no significant main effect of video type [$p = 0.642$]. In neutral conditions, pets were significantly higher than scenery [$p < 0.05$]. Scenery was significantly higher than neutral [$p < 0.01$] (Figure 2).

A repeated-measures ANOVA on emotion valence of video with emotion valence (pet, scenery and neutral) as within-subject variables revealed a significant main effect [$F(2, 70) = 199.894$, $p < 0.001$, $\eta p^2 = 0.851$]. Post hoc tests showed that neutral was significantly lower than that for pet [$p < 0.001$] and scenery [$p < 0.001$]. There was no significant difference between pet and scenery [$p = 0.291$].

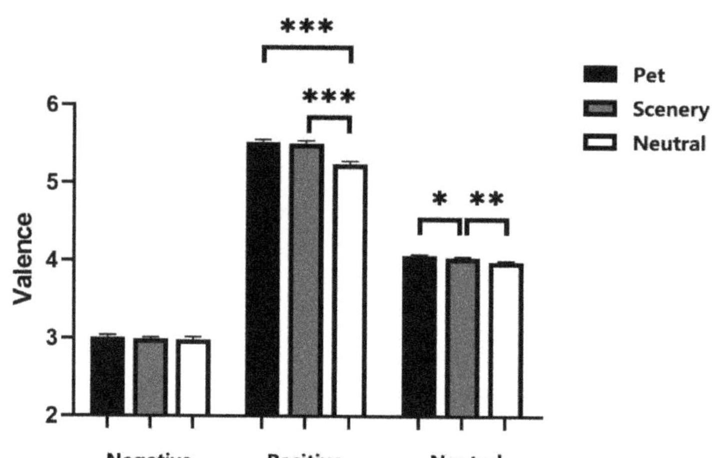

Figure 2. Perceived valence of emotional faces. * $p < 0.05$, ** $p < 0.01$, *** $p < 0.001$. Error bars represent means ± SEM.

https://doi.org/10.3390/ejihpe16020021

To explore whether the change in attentional bias towards positive emotional faces in Experiment 1 was caused by a change in valence perception. A repeated-measures ANOVA on emotion valence with emotion face (positive, neutral) and video type (pet, neutral) as within-subject variables was conducted. The interaction between emotion face and video type was significant [$F(1, 35) = 19.534$, $p < 0.001$, $\eta p^2 = 0.358$]. The disparity between pet stimuli and neutral videos was more pronounced in positive facial expression conditions compared to neutral facial expression conditions.

3.3. Discussion

This study investigated how viewing pet videos influences subsequent perception of facial emotional valence. Results demonstrated that for negative faces, no significant valence differences existed among the three video types. For positive faces, pet and scenery videos exhibited significantly higher valence than neutral videos, with no significant difference between pet and scenery videos. For neutral faces, pet valence was significantly higher than scenery, which was significantly higher than neutral. The participant gave a higher score for the facial valence, indicating that he perceived the face as more positive. Pets exerted a greater influence on valence perception of positive emotional faces compared to neutral ones.

The results of this experiment show that watching emotional videos can significantly influence subsequent valence perception of emotional faces. A recent hypothesis, called the affective realism hypothesis, proposes that affective feelings, as integral properties of individuals' perceptual experiences, akin to experiences of hue and brightness, influence target perception (Anderson et al., 2012; Kring et al., 2014; Gao et al., 2022). Events encountered after an arousing emotional experience may be processed through specific emotional filters, thus "coloring" the perception or evaluation of the event (Grupe et al., 2018). Therefore, the emotions experienced by the participants while watching the video will affect their perception of emotions during the subsequent face processing.

Emotional videos influence various emotional face types distinctly. Positive emotional videos can enhance the valence perception of neutral and positive faces but have no significant effect on negative ones. This might be because negative stimuli hold survival significance (W. Lin et al., 2021), making them less susceptible to influence from other emotional stimuli.

More importantly, pet videos demonstrated specificity in influencing facial emotion perception. For neutral faces, pet videos had a significantly greater impact on emotion perception than scenery videos. This could be attributed to pets' social attributes influencing participants' emotion perception. Xu et al. (2016) used emotionally and socially charged linguistic information as a background to investigate the impact of emotion and sociality on neutral face processing. They discovered that face processing is affected by the interplay of emotion and sociality. In line with previous research, this study suggests that pets' social attributes can specifically influence people's emotional processing of faces with similar attributes.

4. Experiment 3: The Impact of Pet Animal Videos on the Valence Assessment of Emotional Words

The consistent results of Experiment 1 and Experiment 2 demonstrate that pet videos can specifically influence attentional bias toward emotional faces and emotional perception. This effect is likely attributable to the social attributes of pets and faces. If the perception target lacks social attributes, pet videos may not exert specific effects on emotional perception. Consequently, this experiment employs emotional words as the perception target, investigating the impact of emotional videos on valence assessment of emotional words.

https://doi.org/10.3390/ejihpe16020021

Hypothesis 4 was that there was no significant difference in the valence of the positive words, negative words and neutral words among the three conditions.

4.1. Method

4.1.1. Participates

A medium effect size of f = 0.25 was used to conduct a power analysis with G*power 3.1. The estimated sample size needed was at least 34 participants to achieve 80% power and detect the effect given an α level of 0.05. The current experiment recruited 36 college students with normal or corrected-to-normal vision (26 females, aged 21.22 $\pm$ 1.22 years). None of these participants had participated in other experiments from this research.

4.1.2. Experimental Materials

(1) Videos

Same as Experiment 1.

(2) Words

Thirty-two negative words, 32 neutral words, and 32 positive words were selected from the Chinese Affective Words System (Y. Wang et al., 2008). All words were two-character nouns. The text was presented on the screen with a size of 4.5 cm $\times$ 2 cm. The face was located at the center of the screen.

4.1.3. Experimental Procedure

The experimental procedure of Experiment 3 was identical to that of Experiments 1 and 2 in terms of environment, apparatus, and overall design. Participants visited the laboratory on three separate occasions, with intervals of at least three days between sessions, to complete viewing of the three video categories (pet, scenery, and neutral) followed by an emotional word valence evaluation task. The order of video categories was counterbalanced across participants using a Latin square design.

Each session was conducted in a sound-attenuated room, with participants seated 80 cm from the display monitor. The experimental program was implemented using Presentation 0.71 software and presented on a monitor with a refresh rate of 60 Hz.

Each session proceeded as follows. First, participants watched a 10 min silent video corresponding to the assigned condition. Immediately thereafter, they completed an emotional word valence evaluation task. In each trial, a white fixation cross (+) was presented at the center of the screen for 500 ms, followed by the presentation of a two-character emotional word (positive, negative, or neutral), which remained on the screen until a response was made. Participants were instructed to judge the emotional valence of each word as quickly and accurately as possible using numeric keys on the keyboard (1–7; 1 = "most negative," 7 = "most positive"). Upon response, the word disappeared, followed by a randomly jittered blank interval of 1100–1500 ms. The word evaluation task comprised 96 trials presented in random order, including 32 positive, 32 negative, and 32 neutral words.

After completing the task, participants answered two attention-check questions related to the viewed video (e.g., in the pet video condition, "Was Garfield the cat shown in the video?") and rated the emotional valence of the video itself using a 7-point scale (1 = very negative, 7 = very positive).

The experimental environment, phased procedure, video materials, Latin square counterbalancing, and attention-check procedures were strictly identical to those used in Experiments 1 and 2. The primary distinction was that the perceptual targets in Experiment 2 (emotional faces) were replaced with emotional words in the present experiment, allowing

https://doi.org/10.3390/ejihpe16020021

for examination of differences in the effects of pet videos on the processing of social versus non-social emotional stimuli.

4.1.4. Data Analysis

Analyses were performed using SPSS 26.0. The emotional valence of emotional words and videos was analyzed using a repeated-measures ANOVA, with post hoc comparisons conducted using the LSD test and Bonferroni correction applied to adjust for multiple comparisons.

4.2. Results

A repeated-measures ANOVA on emotion valence with emotion word (positive, negative, or neutral) and video type (pet, scenery or neutral) as within-subject variables revealed a significant main effect of emotion word [$F(2, 70) = 711.714$, $p < 0.001$, $\eta p^2 = 0.953$]. There was no significant main effect of video type [$F(2, 70) = 1.967$, $p = 0.147$, $\eta p^2 = 0.053$] or interaction effect [$F(4, 140) = 0.511$, $p = 0.728$, $\eta p^2 = 0.014$] (Figure 3).

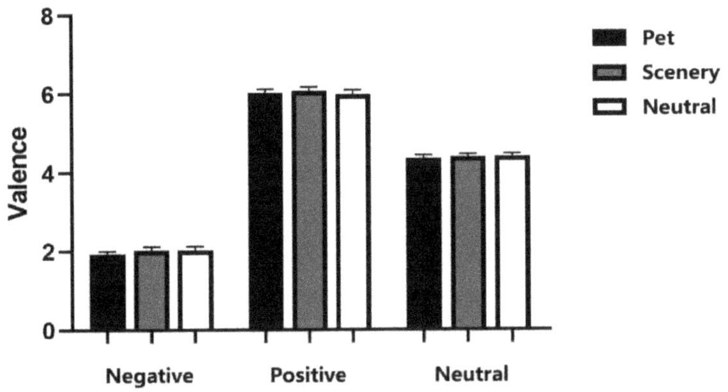

Figure 3. Perceived valence of emotional words. Error bars represent means ± SEM.

A repeated-measures ANOVA on emotion valence of video with emotion valence (pet, scenery and neutral) as within-subject variables revealed a significant main effect [$F(2, 70) = 68.844$, $p < 0.001$, $\eta p^2 = 0.663$]. Post hoc tests showed that neutral was significantly lower than that for pet [$p < 0.001$] and scenery [$p < 0.001$]. There was no significant difference between pet and scenery [$p = 0.133$].

4.3. Discussion

This study investigated how viewing pet videos affected subsequent emotional valence perception of words. The results indicated that none of the videos influenced emotional valence perception.

Numerous studies have demonstrated distinct processing mechanisms between text and images in humans, supported by behavioral (W. Lin et al., 2022) and neuroimaging evidence (Vandenberghe et al., 1996; Reisch et al., 2020; W. Lin et al., 2023). For example, emotional effects elicited by words emerge selectively in late-stage semantic processing, while facial emotional processing dominates early sensory stages (Rellecke et al., 2011; Reisch et al., 2020). Therefore, the valence ratings of emotional words may exhibit lower sensitivity to video-induced modulation compared to facial stimuli.

It should be noted that one of the primary aims of the present experiment was to examine whether the modulatory effect of pet videos on emotional processing depends on the social attributes of the stimuli (e.g., faces used in Experiments 1 and 2). The results showed that pet videos did not modulate the valence perception of non-social emotional

https://doi.org/10.3390/ejihpe16020021

words, suggesting that their effects may be more sensitive to stimuli with social attributes. However, this null effect may also be attributable to systematic differences between words and faces in terms of emotional immediacy, sensory modality, or depth of processing. Future research could further clarify the boundary conditions and cognitive mechanisms underlying the effects of pet videos on emotional processing by directly comparing different types of social and non-social stimuli.

5. General Discussion

This study investigated how pet videos influence emotion processing through three experiments. The results demonstrated that viewing pet videos significantly modulated subsequent attentional bias toward emotional faces by enhancing valence perception of both positive and neutral facial stimuli.

Numerous studies have demonstrated that neural activity and functional connectivity in the brain undergo changes following exposure to emotional stimuli (Eryilmaz et al., 2011; Tambini et al., 2016; Qiao-Tasserit et al., 2024). Tambini et al. (2016) revealed that participants' brains remained emotionally engaged for a period after such exposure, influencing subsequent encoding of emotional stimuli. Some studies even reported increased activity in brain regions such as the anterior cingulate cortex and inferior parietal lobe after watching emotionally charged film clips, compared to activity levels during clip viewing (Eryilmaz et al., 2011). These findings suggest that human emotions and related neural activities remain active for some time after emotional stimulus offset, thereby affecting subsequent cognitive processing. Consequently, the emotional state induced by pet videos did not immediately dissipate but persisted, resulting in altered emotional attention bias and perception in subsequent tasks.

Research findings indicate that pet videos primarily influence emotional face processing by enhancing perceived valence for positive and neutral faces. While Experiment 1 demonstrated that pet videos reduced attentional bias toward negative faces, Experiment 2 revealed this effect was mediated through enhanced valence perception of paired neutral faces, rather than directly influencing attention to negative faces.

In Experiment 2, pet videos enhanced valence perception of both neutral and positive faces, with a significantly stronger enhancement for positive faces compared to neutral ones. Stimuli with higher valence are known to attract greater attentional resources (Carretié et al., 2001). This accounts for why pet videos in Experiment 1 increased participants' attentional bias toward positive faces. This effect may stem from a protective "positivity bias" (Grupe et al., 2018), wherein individuals exhibit heightened sensitivity to positive information. Such a positivity bias has been widely documented across domains, including media (Ng et al., 2023), face processing (Zhao et al., 2017), memory (Ünal & Besken, 2020; Ferguson et al., 2023), and language (Dodds et al., 2014).

Results from Experiments 1–3 demonstrate that pet videos specifically modulate emotional face processing. People primarily keep pets for emotional support (X. Zhang et al., 2024), and media content can produce effects analogous to real-life interactions (Mancuso et al., 2023; Z. Zhang et al., 2024). When viewing pet videos, participants may experience emotional support akin to real-life interactions. Emotional support has been shown to significantly modulate attentional bias toward emotional faces (Dewitte & De Houwer, 2008). Therefore, transient emotional support induced by the videos leads to temporary alterations in emotion processing. However, it should be noted that the present experiment did not directly measure participants' perceived social support while viewing the videos. Therefore, it remains unclear whether the effects of pet videos arise from simulated social support and the fulfillment of affiliation needs, or from a more

 https://doi.org/10.3390/ejihpe16020021

general activation of attentional and affective systems related to living entities. Further investigation is required to disentangle these possibilities.

This study demonstrates that viewing pet videos significantly modulates subsequent emotion processing. Therefore, we propose that the regulatory effects of long-term exposure to pet-related media content on mental health may operate through two distinct pathways.

First, the impact of pet videos on subsequent emotion processing may not be limited to the task period and could last for days or longer. In Grupe et al. (2018), participants were presented with three valence emotional pictures paired with neutral faces. Three days later, their liking and memory for the neutral faces were tested, revealing that both were influenced by the emotional pictures shown three days earlier. The authors suggest that affective information may spill over from preceding and unrelated emotional events in a way that can color the perception or evaluation of unrelated social stimuli. Therefore, regularly watching pet videos may color a large amount of emotional information in people's lives more positively, especially social information, and this positivity can persist in daily life, contributing to better mental health.

Second, the mental health effects of frequent exposure to pet videos may parallel those of positive psychological interventions (PPIs). PPIs are defined as repeated engagement in activities designed to elicit positive emotions, thereby fostering positive emotional states, behaviors, or cognitive patterns in individuals (Sin & Lyubomirsky, 2009), with the ultimate goals of enhancing well-being and alleviating mental disorders. Established PPIs include written positive experiences (Burton & King, 2004), positive future thinking (Peters et al., 2010), and positive self-bias training (L. Wang et al., 2023). The emotional support derived from pets may potentiate the efficacy of such interventions, particularly in enhancing social functioning. It is noteworthy that although the pet videos used in this study were sourced from publicly available online platforms, future applications of such content in formal mental health interventions or research should adhere strictly to non-invasive, animal welfare–oriented ethical guidelines. The production of videos should not pursue human psychological benefits as the sole objective; rather, it should also promote positive human–animal interactions and shared well-being, ensuring that animals remain in a natural, comfortable, and stress-free state throughout recording (Rault et al., 2025). Such practices are not only an ethical requirement for scientific research but also constitute a foundation for developing sustainable and responsible human–animal interactive media.

In summary, long-term exposure to pet videos and images through media may influence mental health via modulation of emotion processing. Our findings provide empirical evidence for elucidating the relationship between media content and human mental health, particularly highlighting the beneficial effects of media-delivered positive information.

This study has several limitations. First, the pet videos used in the experiment lacked real interactions between humans and animals, which limits the extent to which their effects can be directly equated with the social support derived from actual human–animal interactions. Future research should compare the effects of interactive versus non-interactive pet content. Second, we did not assess participants' subjective experience of social support while watching the videos. Future studies could combine such self-report measures with neuroimaging techniques (e.g., fMRI, EEG) to more directly elucidate the underlying cognitive and neural mechanisms. In addition, because participants' pet ownership status was not the primary focus of this study, data regarding this variable were neither collected nor analyzed. Future research could consider including participants' pet ownership and attitudes toward companion animals as potential variables for further investigation. Finally, this study employed a dot-probe task to measure attentional bias. However, it should be noted that the dot-probe task has been widely criticized for its low reliability (Kappenman et al., 2014). Future research could adopt more reliable experimen-

https://doi.org/10.3390/ejihpe16020021

tal paradigms or combine eye-tracking and EEG techniques to validate the present findings and further clarify their cognitive mechanisms. Future investigations could employ longitudinal experimental designs or cognitive neuroscience techniques to further delineate the mechanisms underlying the mental health impacts of chronic media consumption of pet-related content.

6. Conclusions

Our results demonstrate that viewing pet videos decreases attentional bias toward subsequent negative emotional faces while increasing it toward positive ones. This effect stems from enhanced valence perception of subsequent positive and neutral faces. The modulatory effect on emotional faces is specific to pet videos compared to non-social positive ones, attributable to their emotional support properties.

Author Contributions: Conceptualization, W.L.; methodology, W.L.; software, W.L.; formal analysis, W.L.; data curation, X.S.; writing—original draft preparation, X.Z.; writing—review and editing, W.L., J.L. (Jingyuan Lin), J.L. (Jiahao Liang), and B.S.; supervision, W.L. and J.L. (Jingyuan Lin); project administration, W.L. and J.L. (Jingyuan Lin); funding acquisition, W.L. and J.L. (Jingyuan Lin) All authors have read and agreed to the published version of the manuscript.

Funding: This study was supported by the National Natural Science Foundation of China (32400923), the Sichuan Science and Technology Program (2024NSFSC1226) and the Key Projects of Philosophy and Social Sciences (21JZD063).

Institutional Review Board Statement: The study was conducted in accordance with the Declaration of Helsinki and approved by the Ethics Committee of Sichuan Normal University (protocol code 2023LS018 and approval date 15 February 2025).

Informed Consent Statement: Written informed consent was obtained from the participants involved in this study.

Data Availability Statement: The datasets used during the current study are available from the corresponding author.

Conflicts of Interest: The authors declare no competing interests.

References

Anderson, E., Siegel, E., White, D., & Barrett, L. F. (2012). Out of sight but not out of mind: Unseen affective faces influence evaluations and social impressions. *Emotion*, *12*(6), 1210–1221. [CrossRef]

Bowlby, J. A. (2008). *Secure base: Parent-child attachment and healthy human development*. Basic Books.

Brooks, H. L., Rushton, K., Lovell, K., Bee, P., Walker, L., Grant, L., & Rogers, A. (2018). The power of support from companion animals for people living with mental health problems: A systematic review and narrative synthesis of the evidence. *BMC Psychiatry*, *18*, 31. [CrossRef] [PubMed]

Burton, C. M., & King, L. A. (2004). The health benefits of writing about intensely positive experiences. *Journal of Research in Personality*, *38*, 150–163. [CrossRef]

Carretié, L., Mercado, F., Tapia, M., & Hinojosa, J. A. (2001). Emotion, attention, and the 'negativity bias', studied through event-related potentials. *International Journal of Psychophysiology*, *41*, 75–85. [CrossRef]

Cheung, C. K., & Kam, P. K. (2018). Conditions for pets to prevent depression in older adults. *Aging & Mental Health*, *22*, 1627–1633.

Dewitte, M., & De Houwer, J. (2008). Adult attachment and attention to positive and negative emotional face expressions. *Journal of Research in Personality*, *42*(2), 498–505. [CrossRef]

Dodds, P., Clark, E., Desu, S., Frank, M., Reagan, A., Williams, J., Mitchell, L., Harris, K., Kloumann, I., Bagrow, J., Megerdoomian, K., Mcmahon, M., Tivnan, B., & Danforth, C. (2014). Human language reveals a universal positivity bias. *Proceedings of the National Academy of Sciences*, *112*(8), 2389–2394. [CrossRef]

Ein, N., Gervasio, J., Reed, M. J., & Vickers, K. (2023). Effects on wellbeing of exposure to dog videos before a stressor. *Anthrozoös*, *36*(3), 349–367. [CrossRef]

Ein, N., Reed, M. J., & Vickers, K. (2022). The effect of dog videos on subjective and physiological responses to stress. *Anthrozoös*, *35*(3), 463–482. [CrossRef]

https://doi.org/10.3390/ejihpe16020021

Eryilmaz, H., Van De Ville, D., Schwartz, S., & Vuilleumier, P. (2011). Impact of transient emotions on functional connectivity during subsequent resting state: A wavelet correlation approach. *NeuroImage*, *54*(3), 2481–2491. [CrossRef]

Ferguson, L., Harikumar, A., & Leal, S. (2023). Retirement through rose-colored glasses: Greater positivity bias in retired relative to working older adults. *Work, Aging and Retirement*, *11*(2), 162–174. [CrossRef]

Gao, W., Yan, X., & Yuan, J. J. (2022). Neural correlations between cognitive deficits and emotion regulation strategies: Understanding emotion dysregulation in depression from the perspective of cognitive control and cognitive biases. *Psychoradiology*, *2*(3), 86–99. [CrossRef]

Glocker, M. L., Langleben, D. D., Ruparel, K., Loughead, J. W., Gur, R. C., & Sachser, N. (2009). Baby schema in infant faces induces cuteness perception and motivation for caretaking in adults. *Ethology*, *115*(3), 257–263. [CrossRef]

Grupe, D., Schaefer, S., Lapate, R., Schoen, A., Gresham, L., Mumford, J., & Davidson, R. (2018). Behavioral and neural indices of affective coloring for neutral social stimuli. *Social Cognitive and Affective Neuroscience*, *13*(3), 310–320. [CrossRef] [PubMed]

Hajek, A., Peltzer, K., Veronese, N., König, H. H., & Gyasi, R. M. (2024). Pet ownership and psychosocial outcomes among the oldest old in Germany during the COVID-19 pandemic. Findings based on the nationally representative "old age in Germany (D80+)". *International Journal of Geriatric Psychiatry*, *39*(7), e6127. [CrossRef] [PubMed]

Hoagwood, K., Vincent, A., Acri, M., Morrissey, M., Seibel, L., Guo, F., Flores, C., Seag, D., Peth Pierce, R., & Horwitz, S. (2022). Reducing anxiety and stress among youth in a CBT-based equine-assisted adaptive riding program. *Animals*, *12*, 2491. [CrossRef] [PubMed]

Janssens, M., Janssens, E., Eshuis, J., Lataster, J., Simons, M., Reijnders, J., & Jacobs, N. (2021). Companion animals as buffer against the impact of stress on affect: An experience sampling study. *Animals*, *11*, 2171. [CrossRef]

Junça-Silva, A. (2022). Friends with benefits: The positive consequences of pet-friendly practices for workers' well-being. *International Journal of Environmental Research and Public Health*, *19*, 1069. [CrossRef]

Junça-Silva, A., Almeida, M., & Gomes, C. (2022). The role of dogs in the relationship between telework and performance via affect: A moderated moderated mediation analysis. *Animals*, *12*, 1727. [CrossRef]

Kappenman, E. S., Farrens, J. L., Luck, S. J., & Proudfit, G. H. (2014). Behavioral and ERP measures of attentional bias to threat in the dot-probe task: Poor reliability and lack of correlation with anxiety. *Frontiers in Psychology*, *5*, 1368. [CrossRef]

Keefer, L., Landau, M., & Sullivan, D. (2014). Non-human support: Broadening the scope of attachment theory. *Social and Personality Psychology Compass*, *8*(9), 524–535. [CrossRef]

Kogan, L. R., Currin-McCulloch, J., Bussolari, C., Packman, W., & Erdman, P. (2021). The psychosocial influence of companion animals on positive and negative affect during the COVID-19 pandemic. *Animals*, *11*, 2084. [CrossRef] [PubMed]

Kring, A. M., Siegel, E. H., & Barrett, L. F. (2014). Unseen affective faces influence person perception judgments in schizophrenia. *Clinical Psychological Science*, *2*(4), 443–454. [CrossRef] [PubMed]

Langston, S. C. (2014). *Understanding and quantifying the roles of perceived social support, pet attachment, and adult attachment in adult pet owners' sense of well-being* [Doctoral dissertation, Washington State University].

Lavan, S., Ein, N., & Vickers, K. (2023). Examining the effects of nature and animal videos on stress. *Anthrozoös*, *36*(5), 849–868. [CrossRef]

Li, S., Lin, W., Chen, J., & Mo, L. (2025). Psychological benefits of companion animals: Exploring the distinction between ownership and online animal watching. *Society & Animals*, *1*(aop), 1–21. [CrossRef]

Li, Y., Zhang, D., Liu, X., & Guo, D. (2024). Processing facial emojis as social information: Evidence from visual working memory for facial emojis, simple shapes, human faces, and their relations to theory of mind. *Computers in Human Behavior*, *153*, 108106. [CrossRef]

Lin, J., Yang, X., Li, H., Lin, W., Zhang, J., & Lei, Y. (2024). Enhancing agency in individuals with depressive symptoms: The roles of effort, outcome valence, and its underlying cognitive mechanisms and neural basis. *Depression and Anxiety*, *2024*, 3135532. [CrossRef]

Lin, W., Li, Z., Zhang, X., Gao, Y., & Lin, J. (2023). Electrophysiological evidence for the effectiveness of images versus text in warnings. *Scientific Reports*, *13*, 1278. [CrossRef] [PubMed]

Lin, W., Lin, J., Li, Z., Wei, R., Cai, X., & Mo, L. (2021). Different effects of feedback-induced emotion and material-induced emotion on memory. *Psychological Research*, *85*, 2530–2537. [CrossRef]

Lin, W., Lin, J., Yang, Y., Liao, J., Chen, W., & Mo, L. (2022). The difference in the warning effect of different warning signs. *International Journal of Occupational Safety and Ergonomics*, *28*(2), 890–900. [CrossRef]

Lisa, Z., Kipling, D. W., & Rick, R. (2004). How low can you go? Ostracism by a computer is sufficient to lower self-reported levels of belonging, control, self-esteem, and meaningful existence. *Journal of Experimental Social Psychology*, *40*(4), 560–567.

Liu, H., Lin, J., & Lin, W. (2024). Cognitive mechanisms and neurological foundations of companion animals' role in enhancing human psychological well-being. *Frontiers in Psychology*, *15*, 1354220. [CrossRef] [PubMed]

Liu, H., Zhou, X., Lin, J., & Lin, W. (2025). Specific neural mechanisms underlying humans' processing of information related to companion animals: A comparison with domestic animals and objects. *Animals*, *15*(21), 3162. [CrossRef]

 https://doi.org/10.3390/ejihpe16020021

MacLeod, C., & Clarke, P. (2015). The attentional bias modification approach to anxiety intervention. *Clinical Psychological Science*, *3*(1), 58–78. [CrossRef]

MacLeod, C., & Mathews, A. (1988). Anxiety and the allocation of attention to threat. *The Quarterly Journal of Experimental Psychology A: Human Experimental Psychology*, *40*(4), 653–670. [CrossRef] [PubMed]

Mancuso, V., Bruni, F., Stramba-Badiale, C., Riva, G., Cipresso, P., & Pedroli, E. (2023). How do emotions elicited in virtual reality affect our memory? A systematic review. *Computers in Human Behavior*, *146*, 107812. [CrossRef]

Mormann, F., Dubois, J., Kornblith, S., Milosavljevic, M., Cerf, M., Ison, M., Tsuchiya, N., Kraskov, A., Quiroga, R. Q., Adolphs, R., & Fried, I. (2011). A category-specific response to animals in the right human amygdala. *Nature Neuroscience*, *14*(10), 1247–1249. [CrossRef]

Myrick, J. G. (2015). Emotion regulation, procrastination, and watching cat videos online: Who watches internet cats, why, and to what effect? *Computers in Human Behavior*, *52*, 168–176. [CrossRef]

Na, H., & Dong, S. Y. (2023). Mixed-reality-based human-animal interaction can relieve mental stress. *Frontiers in Veterinary Science*, *10*, 1102937. [CrossRef]

Ng, Z. Z., Li, G., Flynn, S., & Yow, W. Q. (2023). How COVID-19 news affect older adults' mental health—Evidence of a positivity bias. *International Journal of Environmental Research and Public Health*, *20*(5), 3950. [CrossRef]

Peters, M. L., Flink, I. K., Boersma, K., & Linton, S. J. (2010). Manipulating optimism: Can imagining a best possible self be used to increase positive future expectancies? *Journal of Positive Psychology*, *5*(3), 204–211. [CrossRef]

Posner, M. I., & Petersen, S. E. (1990). The attention system of the human brain. *Annual Review of Neuroscience*, *13*, 25–42. [CrossRef]

Qiao-Tasserit, E., Corradi-Dell'Acqua, C., & Vuilleumier, P. (2024). Influence of transient emotional episodes on affective and cognitive theory of mind. *Social Cognitive and Affective Neuroscience*, *19*, nsae016. [CrossRef]

Quan, W., Kim, S., Baah, N. G., Jung, H., & Han, H. (2023). Role of physical environment and green natural environment of pet-accompanying tourism sites in generating pet owners' life satisfaction. *Journal of Travel & Tourism Marketing*, *40*(5), 399–415. [CrossRef]

Rathish, D., Rajapakse, J., & Weerakoon, K. (2022). "In times of stress, it is good to be with them": Experience of dog owners from a rural district of Sri Lanka. *BMC Public Health*, *22*, 2380. [CrossRef] [PubMed]

Rault, J. L., Bateson, M., Boissy, A., Forkman, B., Grinde, B., Gygax, L., Harfeld, J. L., Hintze, S., Keeling, L. J., Kostal, L., & Lawrence, A. B. (2025). A consensus on the definition of positive animal welfare. *Biology Letters*, *21*(1), 20240382. [CrossRef]

Reisch, L. M., Wegrzyn, M., Woermann, F. G., Bien, C. G., & Kissler, J. (2020). Negative content enhances stimulus-specifc cerebral activity during free viewing of pictures, faces, and words. *Human Brain Mapping*, *41*(15), 4332–4354. [CrossRef]

Rellecke, J., Palazova, M., Sommer, W., & Schacht, A. (2011). On the automaticity of emotion processing in words and faces: Event-related brain potentials evidence from a superficial task. *Brain and Cognition*, *77*(1), 23–32. [CrossRef]

Shearer, A., Hunt, M., Chowdhury, M., & Nicol, L. (2016). Effects of a brief mindfulness meditation intervention on student stress and heart rate variability. *International Journal of Stress Management*, *23*, 232–254. [CrossRef]

Si, H., Yu, F., Lee, T. M., & Li, Z. (2025). Millions of pet videos deepen our understanding of human–cat interactions with implications for management. *People and Nature*, *7*, 2228–2240. [CrossRef]

Sin, N. L., & Lyubomirsky, S. (2009). Enhancing well-being and alleviating depressive symptoms with positive psychology interventions: A practice-friendly meta-analysis. *Journal of Clinical Psychology*, *65*(5), 467–487. [CrossRef]

Tambini, A., Rimmele, U., Phelps, E. A., & Davachi, L. (2016). Emotional brain states carry over and enhance future memory formation. *Nature Neuroscience*, *20*(2), 271. [CrossRef] [PubMed]

Taylor, P., Ditommaso, E., Scott-Storey, K., O'Donnell, S., Busolo, D., Vincent, C. D., & Malcolm, J. (2024). Attachment, mental health, and alcohol use by men: The mediating role of cumulative lifetime violence severity. *American Journal of Men's Health*, *18*(5), 15579883241293293. [CrossRef]

Ünal, B., & Besken, M. (2020). Blessedly forgetful and blissfully unaware: A positivity bias in memory for (re)constructions of imagined past and future events. *Memory*, *28*, 888–899. [CrossRef] [PubMed]

Vandenberghe, R., Price, C., Wise, R., Josephs, O., & Frackowiak, R. S. (1996). Functional anatomy of a common semantic system for words and pictures. *Nature*, *383*(6597), 254–256. [CrossRef]

Wang, L., Song, X., Jia, F., Xue, W., & Li, L. (2023). Effectiveness of enhanced self-positivity bias training in mitigating depressive mood following negative life events. *Behavioral Sciences*, *13*(7), 534. [CrossRef]

Wang, Y., & Luo, Y. (2005). Standardization and assessment of college students' facial expression of emotion. *Chinese Journal of Clinical Psychology*, *13*(4), 396–398.

Wang, Y., Zhou, L., & Luo, Y. (2008). The pilot establishment and evaluation of Chinese affective words system. *Chinese Mental Health Journal*, *8*, 608–612.

Wei, Z., Guo, Y., Tsang, M. H. L., Montag, C., Becker, B., & Kou, J. (2024). Social media distractions alter behavioral and neural patterns to global-local attention: The moderation effect of fear of missing out. *Computers in Human Behavior*, *157*, 108258. [CrossRef]

Wells, D. L. (2019). The state of research on human–animal relations: Implications for human health. *Anthrozoos*, *32*(2), 169–181. [CrossRef]

Wilson, E. O. (1984). *Biophilia*. Harvard University Press.

Xu, M., Li, Z., Diao, L., Fan, L., & Yang, D. (2016). Contextual valence and sociality jointly influence the early and later stages of neutral face processing. *Frontiers in Psychology*, *7*, 1258. [CrossRef]

Yang, J., Zhou, L., & Hu, Z. (2024). Social excluder's face reduces gaze-triggered attention orienting. *Psychological Research*, *88*(4), 1352–1361. [CrossRef]

Yang, M., Zhang, L., Zhang, P., Wei, Z., Xu, L., Huang, L., Kendrick, K., Lei, Y., & Kou, J. (2024). Neural and gaze pattern responses to happy faces in autism: Predictors of adaptive difficulties and re-evaluation of the social motivation hypothesis. *International Journal of Clinical and Health Psychology*, *24*(4), 100527. [CrossRef] [PubMed]

Zhang, X., He, Y., Yang, S., & Wang, D. (2024). Human preferences for dogs and cats in China: The current situation and influencing factors of watching online videos and pet ownership. *Animals*, *14*, 3458. [CrossRef] [PubMed]

Zhang, Z., Niu, P., Li, C., & Feng, Y. (2024). Does using a green gaming system make people more environmentally friendly? *Computers in Human Behavior*, *161*, 108392. [CrossRef]

Zhao, S., Xiang, Y., Xie, J., Ye, Y., Li, T., & Mo, L. (2017). The positivity bias phenomenon in face perception given different information on ability. *Frontiers in Psychology*, *8*, 570. [CrossRef]

Zhou, X., & Shen, X. (2024). Unveiling the relationship between social anxiety, loneliness, motivations, and problematic smartphone use: A network approach. *Comprehensive Psychiatry*, *130*, 152451. [CrossRef]

https://doi.org/10.3390/ejihpe16020021

MDPI AG
Grosspeteranlage 5
4052 Basel
Switzerland
Tel.: +41 61 683 77 34

European Journal of Investigation in Health, Psychology and Education Editorial Office
E-mail: ejihpe@mdpi.com
www.mdpi.com/journal/ejihpe

www.ingramcontent.com/pod-product-compliance
Lightning Source LLC
Chambersburg PA
CBHW062044220926
51850CB00010B/2662